The Institute of Biology's
Studies in Biology no. 152

Malaria

R.S. Phillips

Senior Lecturer in Zoology,
University of Glasgow

Edward Arnold

First published 1983
by Edward Arnold (Publishers) Limited
41 Bedford Square, London WC1 3DQ

ISBN 0–7131–2858–5

Printed and bound in Great Britain at
The Camelot Press Ltd, Southampton

General Preface to the Series

Because it is no longer possible for one textbook to cover the whole field of biology while remaining sufficiently up to date, the Institute of Biology proposed this series so that teachers and students can learn about significant developments. The enthusiastic acceptance of 'Studies in Biology' shows that the books are providing authoritative views of biological topics.

The features of the series include the attention given to methods, the selected list of books for further reading and, wherever possible, suggestions for practical work.

Readers' comments will be welcomed by the Education Officer of the Institute.

1983   Institute of Biology
                                                         20 Queensbury Place
                                                         London SW7 2DZ

Preface

The aims of this book are two-fold. First I hope it will provide a basic grounding in the study of malaria, to which a more detailed knowledge of the subject may be added later. If along the way some readers are fired with sufficient enthusiasm to pursue a career in any aspect of malaria and malaria parasites, the second aim will have been achieved. Malaria is still the most important tropical disease of man and as such presents a major challenge. A significant development in meeting this challenge is that those involved are not, as in the past, primarily drawn from the ranks of the entomologists and clinicians, both of whom still play major roles, but now immunologists, biochemists, geneticists and others are bringing their expertise to bear on the problem of malaria.

Acknowledgements My colleagues, Graham Coombs, Kathleen Harvey, John Kusel, and Sheila McLean, read and made useful comments on different sections of the manuscript. Dr R.E. Sinden provided the electron micrographs. Miss T. Emerson and Mrs M. McCulloch typed the manuscript. I thank all these people most warmly.

Glasgow, 1983   R.S.P.

Contents

1 Introduction

In 1956 the World Health Organisation (WHO) initiated its major campaign to rid the world of malaria. This campaign was not based on the use of an effective vaccine, as was the highly successful WHO campaign which has led to the eradication of smallpox, but primarily on the use of the cheap, and then effective, residual insecticide DDT. This was employed, along with other measures, to reduce the numbers of the vector of the malaria parasite, the female anopheline mosquito, and hence to interrupt transmission of malaria. Initially the list of areas where control and eradication measures were successful lengthened. So successful did the campaign appear to be that a popular British daily newspaper in its leader in September 1978 stated that 'malaria had been wiped out'. Nothing could be further from the truth. Although areas such as the United States, much of Europe, Israel and Cyprus are now free of indigenous malaria, in parts of the tropics, especially tropical Africa, control measures, where used, have made little impact on the disease. In the Indian subcontinent an impressive reduction in the number of cases of malaria was achieved by the early 1960s, but over the past five years there has been a disastrous resurgence in the disease. In India in 1966 about 40 000 cases of malaria were reported: in 1976, 5.8 million were reported and it is estimated that in 1977 there were at least 10 million cases. Similar disturbing rises in malaria cases are reported in Central America. The reasons why malaria remains a serious and increasing problem are several. Some mosquitoes are resistant to insecticides, some parasites are resistant to anti-malarial drugs, and social and economic pressures have conspired to prevent governments from implementing or maintaining effective control schemes. WHO estimate that in 1976 352 million people were living in areas with no specific anti-malarial measures and since 1971 there had been a two-fold increase in reported cases. Malaria still exists in about 100 countries; in many parts of Africa, Central and South America, Asia and the Pacific. In Africa alone 1 million people, mainly infants and children, die annually from malaria. Almost 100 years after Laveran became the first man to see the malaria parasite in the blood of a soldier, this parasite remains one of the greatest single killers of man. Such is the gravity of the malaria problem in some countries, that not only is the health of the population threatened, but also the social and economic development of the communities.

Malaria and malaria parasites therefore demand attention because of their effects on the health of so many. Biologists, chemists, clinicians, health service administrators and others are all involved in the renewal of efforts to combat the disease, and this booklet in part attempts to explain the role these individuals may be playing. Malaria parasites are, however, also of intrinsic biological interest in themselves. They are protozoans. Their life cycle is complex, involving a vertebrate host and the female mosquito. During this life cycle they may be intracellular, occupying at different times fixed tissue cells or erythrocytes, or they may be extracellular, albeit very briefly. The parasites therefore must have a versatile metabolic system. They change their form and they have an ability to recognize, enter and leave the type of cells appropriate for each stage in their life cycle. They must be able to survive the attempts of the defence system of the vertebrate host to remove them long enough to allow transmission to the next host to occur. A well-known characteristic of malaria infections is their longevity.

Malaria parasites are found in birds, mammals, and lizards, each species having evolved a close relationship with its particular vertebrate host. Correspondingly each species of malaria parasite tends to be specific to one or a few species of vertebrate host: the malaria parasites of man will not grow and develop in rodents but only in man and a limited range of monkeys. Although observations have been made on human malaria parasites in naturally-infected patients, infected volunteers and patients in the advanced stages of syphilis (in whom malaria infections are deliberately initiated as part of the treatment for their spirochaete infection), much of our knowledge of the biology, immunology and biochemistry of malaria parasites has come from studies on animal malarias in laboratory animals. In this book the emphasis will be on our knowledge of human malarias, but it will be supplemented from the vast literature in animal malarias when required.

The goal of most malariologists is to contribute directly or indirectly to the further control and perhaps eventual eradication of the disease, be this through the control of mosquitoes, using chemical or biological methods, or anti-parasitic measures, involving the use of anti-malarial drugs or a malarial vaccine or a combination of both. A greater insight into any aspect of malaria parasites and malaria infections will contribute to this although this may not be immediately apparent. The study of malaria has moved a long way from the days when its investigation was the preoccupation of the army or colonial medical man. In 1976 $80 million was allocated for cancer research in the United States alone but only $40 million world-wide towards research on tropical diseases. The aim of this book is to introduce the topic of malaria and to emphasize that the causative agent is a parasite of great interest, and importance which, perhaps most significantly, is still presenting a challenge worth accepting.

2 A History of Malaria

Malaria ('bad air') is recorded in writings from ancient times. References to the fever, the well-known symptom of malaria, are made in papyri from ancient Egypt. Hippocrates was the first to describe the disease in detail. Therefore the effects of the disease were frequently described although the causative agent was not recognized until close on a century ago. In particular the influence of malaria on military campaigns is referred to time and again. Malaria associated with the marshy Campagna Romana repulsed invaders of ancient Rome better than the weapons of its defenders. The same malarious area accounted for about 8000 victims nearly 2000 years later, in 1944, before the battle for Cassino. Indeed there were as many cases of malaria as there were battle casualities in a number of areas during the second World War. More recently the loss from active service of military personnel due to malaria was the most important single problem the U.S. army faced in the late 1960s in Vietnam.

Discovery of a treatment for malaria fortunately was not as long delayed as the discovery of the cause of the disease. At the beginning of the seventeenth century Amerindians in Peru were using the bark of the tree, which was subsequently named Cinchona, as a cure for malaria. This treatment was given successfully to the malarious wife of the Spanish Viceroy of Peru, the Countess of Chinchon, in 1629, and she took some of the bark back to Spain with her 11 years later. The beneficial properties of the bark became known in Spain, and from there the bark passed to other parts of Europe. Jesuits in Rome apparently carried out the first experiments in anti-malarial chemotherapy with the cinchona bark·powder. The powder became known as Jesuits' or Countess' powder. The cinchona tree in the nineteenth century was established in India, Ceylon and the East Indies. The most important active principal in the bark, the alkaloid quinine, was extracted by the French chemist, Pelletier, in 1820. Thereafter quinine was widely used.

From early times 'ague' or malaria, as the disease became known, was associated with marshes. Indeed paludism, as malaria is also known, is from the French word for a swamp or marsh. In Italy drainage of swamps as a method of controlling the incidence of the disease was practised from the early seventeenth century. It was commonly thought that the agent responsible for the disease wafted in the air emanating from these wet areas. The first important step towards identifying the true cause of the disease is attributed to Meckel, a German pathologist, who realized in 1847 that the black granules he saw in the blood, spleen and liver of cadavers were associated with malaria infections. As we shall see later, the parasite within the red blood cell digests haemoglobin from which it derives amino acids and at the same time produces an insoluble waste product called haemozoin. The black brown pigment is easily seen in the mature parasite in the red cell. When the infected red cell bursts the pigment is released and is subsequently picked up by phagocytic cells in the blood, spleen and liver. The black granules Meckel saw were malaria pigment. Nearly 30 years later, Kelsch, a French pathologist, working in Algerian hospitals looked at fresh blood from malaria patients under the microscope. He noted, as his predecessors did, the presence of pigment in the blood but for the first time he observed that pigment was most noticeable just before the patient became feverish. This, if he did but know it, indicated that he had been looking at parasitized red cells/The crucial finding that not only pigment but also the parasite itself was present in the blood from these patients was made by another French pathologist, Laveran. Laveran, a military doctor like his famous contemporary, Ronald Ross, was sent to Algeria in 1878. He too, examined fresh blood from malarious patients and saw leucocytes (white cells) containing pigment as others had described but he also saw clear bodies which contained pigment. These clear bodies were of two shapes, spheres and crescents, and he suspectd they were parasites. Confirmation came on 6th November 1880, when he saw in the blood of a young soldier, whose blood was rich in crescents, the process now known as exflagellation. These crescents are the sexual forms of the malaria parasite *Plasmodium falciparum,* and during exflagellation the male crescent rounds up and throws out filaments, or flagella, which detach themselves and, as male gametes, are ready to fertilize the female gametes)

Without the excitement of seeing this process at first hand, Laveran's contemporaries in the scientific and medical community were sceptical: seeing was indeed believing. Only a year before Laveran's discovery two Italians, Klebs and Tommasi-Crudeli, had claimed finding a bacillus in the marshes of a malarious area which could produce symptoms of malaria in rabbits. This was at the time that Pasteur and Koch were formulating the 'germ' theory of disease and hence an association of malaria with a bacillus was taken seriously, with a consequent neglect of Laveran's report. In due course, however, Laveran was vindicated. The Italians, Marchiafava and Celli, working together, in 1884 and 1885, saw the asexual multiplicative forms in the red cells of patients. Another Italian, Golgi, made the significant observation that after the parasite had divided in the red cell the products of this division (merozoites) are released with the bursting of the red cell and that the parasites in separate red cells were all released at about the same time. Fever followed soon after the bursting of the red cells. About the same time, Danilewsky, a Russian working in Kharkov, independently found malaria parasites in frogs and birds.

The cause of malaria had been discovered and its behaviour in the red blood cells of patients and birds observed. The next step forward, that made by Ronald Ross, with the encouragement of Patrick Manson, was in pinpointing the role of the female mosquito. Folklore in several parts of the world had malaria and mosquitoes somehow associated. Laveran himself thought this. Manson, working in China, in the late 1870s showed that mosquitoes might be vectors of filarial worms, the parasites which can cause the gross deformities of the body known as elephantiasis. In 1894 and 1896 he speculated on a similar role for the mosquito in the spread of malaria; the speculation was supported by the knowledge that earlier, in 1893, Smith and Kilbourne had published their classic experiments which demonstrated for the first time that an arthropod (a tick) could transmit a protozoan, in this case, *Babesia,* a parasite of the red blood cells of cattle. Ross and Manson began their association in 1894 when Ross was home on leave from India. In 1895 Ross returned to India to study the malaria parasite in the mosquito. For two years he dissected mosquitoes which had been fed on malarious patients, but in vain because, unknown to him, he was working with the wrong mosquitoes. June 1897, in Secunderbad, saw a change in Ross' fortunes and his perseverance was rewarded. By chance at last the right kind of mosquitoes, 'the dapple-winged' *Anopheles* were brought to him (later identified as *A. stephensi*) and 4 to 5 days after feeding them on infected patients he recognized, in the stomach of two of the mosquitoes, specks of black pigment which revealed the presence of the malaria parasite. This was on August 20th, 1897. His finding was published in the *Lancet* on December 18th, 1897. Shortly after Ross made his discovery he left Secunderbad and further work on human malaria was not possible. The following year he resumed his investigations, perforce on a malaria parasite of sparrows. By July 1898 he found that the infective stages of the malaria parasite *(Plasmodium relictum)* eventually appear in the salivary gland of the mosquito and that, by feeding mosquitoes with these parasites (sporozoites) in their salivary glands on healthy sparrows, the malaria infection could be passed on. The role of the mosquito as the vector of malaria had been demonstrated at last. Confirmation of a similar cycle (sporogonic cycle) for the human malaria parasites, *P. falciparum* and *P. vivax* in *Anopheles claviger*, was published by Italian workers in November and December of the same year. In their report the Italians made passing scant reference to Ross' work, thereby precipitating a lifelong dispute between one of them, Grassi, and Ross over who was first to trace the development of the malaria parasite in the mosquito. Ross was not aware, nor were the Italians, of what happened during the first few hours of the malaria parasite's life in the mosquito's midgut, i.e. the maturation of the sexual forms and fertilization of the female gamete to form a motile zygote (ookinete) which burrows through the gut wall. In fact, fertilization had seen and described in 1897 by MacCallum in Ontario, albeit in a near relative of the malaria parasites, *Haemoproteus columbiae,* in pigeons. The significance of MacCallum's observations was not appreciated by his contemporaries.

Grassi in 1902 speculated that there must be an occult phase in the life of the malaria parasite between the sporozoite being introduced by the female mosquito and the parasite subsequently entering a red blood cell. Soon after this, the eminent biologist, Schaudin, described seeing sporozoites of *P. vivax* entering red cells and such was his reputation that his observations were accepted as true and the search for the occult phase was not pursued. Thirty years later Raffaele (1934) described asexual multiplication (schizogony) of the bird malaria parasite *P. elongatum,* in the reticulo-endothelial cells of the bone marrow and internal organs. A cycle of development outside the red cell (i.e. an exoerythrocytic cycle) was recognized. That a tissue phase also interceded between the sporozoite and the red cell phases in mammalian malaria was demonstrated fi.st by Garnham in 1947 in *Hepatocystis kochi*, a near relative of *Plasmodium*, and secondly by Short and Garnham and their collaborators in 1948 in *Plasmodium*. The tissue was the liver and the phase in the liver was described first for the monkey *Plasmodium, P. cynomolgi,* and later, with the aid of voluteers, for *P. vivax* and *P. falciparum,* parasites of man. The basic cycle of the malaria parasite in all its complexities had been elucidated at last. In the next chapter, this life cycle will be examined in more detail.

3 Morphology and Life Cycles

3.1 Classification and evolution

The details of the classifiction of malaria parasites are, to some extent, a matter of opinion. We shall use that of Baker which is as follows: Malaria parasites are in the Phylum Sporozoa (all parasitic and typically have a resistant spore or a stage derived from the spore and contain sporozoites), Class Telosporea (sexual reproduction and sporozoites in all), Sub-Class Coccidia (mature tropozoites small and intracellular), Order Eucoccida (schizogony, asexual and sexual reproduction) and Sub-order Haemosporina (two hosts, sexual reproduction completed in dipterous insect, asexual development in vertebrate). Included in the Haemosporina along with the malaria parasite *Plasmodium*, are *Hepatocystis* and *Haemoproteus*.

The evolution of the malaria parasites can only be speculative. Gregarines, parasites of invertebrates, appear to be the basic sporozoan stock. The immediate sporozoan ancestors of plasmodia are thought by some to be single host parasites of vertebrates and by others parasites of invertebrates. Within the Haemosporina *Plasmodium* probably evolved most recently. The plasmodia of reptiles and birds separated from those of mammals early in their evolution. The evolution of the mammalian plasmodia probably followed that of the mammals, which would place the primate malaria parasites as the most recent. It is thought that the quartan plasmodia (e.g. *P. inui* and *P. malariae*) are the oldest and *P. falciparum* one of the youngest.

The malaria parasites of mammals and birds are transmitted by female anopheline and culcine mosquitoes respectively. The vector of reptilian malarias has not been determined. It is likely it will prove to be a culcine mosquito, although phlebotomines (sand-flies) have also been suggested. In describing the life cycle of *Plasmodium* (Fig. 3–1) we will concentrate on the malaria parasites of mammals and for comparison summarize the differences we see between them and the avian malarias. In concluding this section a brief description will be given of the malaria parasites of man and of those parasites which are frequently used in experimental work.

3.2 Life cycle

3.2.1 Sporozoites and liver stages in the mammalian host

The infected female mosquito is attracted to her prey and in taking her blood meal the mosquito releases into the capillary bed of the skin saliva containing sporozoites. These are haltere shaped (Fig. 3–2b), around 11 μm in length and 1 μm in diameter and are motile. With the electron microscope, the sporozoites are seen (Fig. 3–2a) to have a surface or pellicle consisting of two

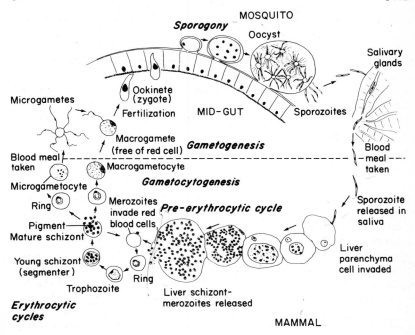

Fig. 3–1 The life cycle of a mammalian *Plasmodium*.

membranes, and below this rows of microtubules, running longitudinally. At the anterior end of the sporozoite are the organelles, collectively known as the apical complex, which are associated with penetration of cells and are seen in other invasive stages in the life cycle (Fig. 3–1) of the parasite. This apical complex consists of polar rings, several long rhoptries, many micronemes and sometimes a collar. The sporozoites enter the blood-stream via the capillaries in the skin and within 30–60 minutes are cleared from the circulation.

Recent investigations suggest that the sporozoite may associate with the phagocytic Kuppfer cell in the liver, en route to the liver parenchyma cell, or hepatocyte, after being introduced by the mosquito. How the sporozoite recognizes and enters the hepatocyte is not known, nor are details of its very early development. Within the hepatocyte the parasite, now known as the pre- or exo-erythrocytic schizont, lies within a vacuole (parasitophorous vacuole) in the host cell cytoplasm and is surrounded by two membranes. The nutrition of the parasite in the hepatocyte is unknown but presumably involves diffusion and pinocytosis. There is no cytostome (mouth). The schizont grows and the vacuole comes to fill most of an enlarged hepatocyte. The nucleus divides many times and the nuclei are distributed through the as yet undivided cytoplasm. As the schizont matures the cytoplasm becomes divided into pseudocytomeres and the nuclei line up along their periphery. Individual parasites, merozoites, are then formed by a process of budding (Fig. 3–2A). Apical rings and rhoptries form in the bud, a nucleus enters it and the merozoites (Fig. 3–2A) so formed detach from the remaining residual body. Rupture of the infected hepatocyte releases thousands of merozoites (Fig. 3–1). The period taken for this pre-erythrocytic cycle to be completed depends on the species of *Plasmodium*. For example a rodent malaria, *P. berghei*, requires about 51 hours whereas the human malaria, *P. vivax*, takes just over 8 days.

3.2.2   The erythrocytic stages

The pear-shaped merozoites are about 1.5 μm in length (Fig. 3–2A, 3–2B), have a double-membraned pellicle plus a plasma membrane carrying a surface coat, an apical complex, a nucleus, a non-functioning cytostome, ribosomes and smooth concentric membranes. The polar rings in the apical complex are thought to be important in maintaining the shape of the apical or anterior prominence. The merozoites released into the blood must survive this temporary extracellular situation while it recognizes and attaches to the red cells. For the mammalian malarias at least it is now thought unlikely that, in any species, merozoites emanating from hepatocytes invade further hepatocytes. On the surface of the merozoite is a surface coat consisting of fine filaments sticking out like bristles, by means of which the merozoite adheres to the red cell surface. Invasion is only initiated if the parasite sticks to the red cell by the apical end (Fig. 3–2A). If invasion is not initiated merozoites can detach. Attachment appears to be dependent on specific red cell receptors, the nature of which is not certain (see Chapter 7). Following attachment, material is thought to be released from the rhoptries and micronemes in the apical complex causing a rapid invagination of the red cell surface. A cavity forms in the cytoplasm of the red cell, which cuts off from the surface of the red cell and encloses the parasite. The invasion process takes no longer than a minute. The cavity (parasitophorous vacuole) containing the parasite is, therefore, lined with a membrane derived from the surface of the red cell. In invading the red cell the merozoite appears to shed its surface coat into the plasma. The merozoite now rapidly transforms into the feeding or trophozoite stage (Fig. 3–2B) and in blood smears stained with Giemsa's stain the parasite appears vacuolated and is referred to as a ring stage. The vacuolar area is probably continuous with the host cell cytoplasm and represents invaginations of the parasite surface. Rhoptries and micronemes have disappeared. The cytostome becomes functional, and host cytoplasm is ingested and is partially digested in membrane lined vesicles known as phagosomes (Fig. 3–2B). Digestion of haemoglobin is incomplete and crystalline granules of pigment or haemozoin are left as a waste product. The parasite enlarges, loses its vacuolar appearance, and fills most or all of the red cell. Division or schizogony now occurs. The nucleus apparently divides repeatedly by mitosis and nuclear fission, the nuclear membrane remaining intact during the division processes. The number of nuclei formed is between 8 and 24 per schizont depending on

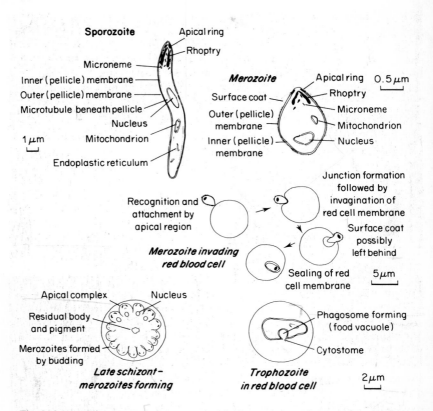

Fig. 3–2 (A) Diagrammatic appearance of the fine structure of some of the stages in the life cycle of *Plasmodium*.

the species of *Plasmodium*. As in the pre-erythrocytic schizont, merozoites are formed by a process of budding which occurs just below the surface membrane, the plasmalemma, of the parasite. Polar rings form within the developing bud, while other organelles, such as rhoptries and micronemes, differentiate in the cytoplasm of the developing schizont and pass into the bud. A nucleus finally passes into each bud, and the fully formed merozoite detaches from the remaining cytoplasm or residual body of the parent cell. The residual body also contains the pigment which on release is rapidly phagocytosed by macrophages, particularly in the liver and spleen. The red cell ruptures by an unknown process releasing the merozoites which invade further red cells (Fig. 3–1). The asexual process can be repeated many times and the blood parasitaemia rises. The time taken to complete the asexual cycle depends on the species of malaria parasite but it is usually 24, 48 or 72 hours. The avian malaria *P. gallinaceum* is unusual in that the asexual cycle takes 36 hours.

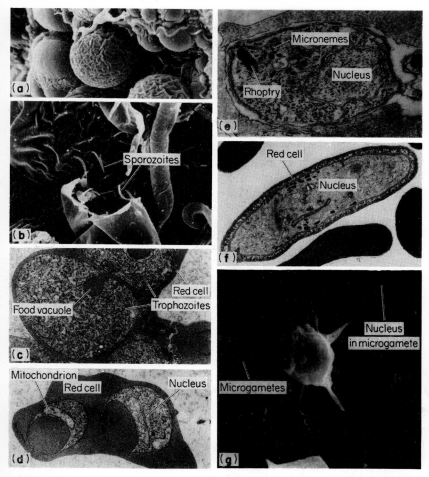

(B) Electron micrographs illustrating the fine structure of *Plasmodium*. (a) Scanning electron micrograph (SEM) of Day 7 oocyst (× 1100): **(b)** SEM of Day 12 oocyst releasing sporozoites (× 1200): **(c)** Trophozoites showing cytoplasm dotted with ribosomes on endoplasmic reticulum (× 1800): **(d)** Ring stages (× 1400): **(e)** LS merozoite in mature schizont (× 56,000): **(f)** Macrogametocyte of *P. falciparum* (×19,000): **(g)** SEM of exflagellation (× 9000).

Certain merozoites from pre-erythrocytic (in some rodent malarias at least) or erythrocytic schizonts are destined to undergo gametocytogenesis, i.e. to differentiate into the sexual stages or gametocytes within the red cells. The stimulus or trigger which directs a merozoite into the sexual rather than the asexual cycle is not known: undefined factors in plasma, loss of CO_2, pH changes, HCO_3^- ions have been implicated. Early in the development of gametocytes their morphological appearance in stained blood smears may be similar to that of growing trophozoites. When they reach maturity, however, and occupy the entire volume of the cell their morphology easily distinguishes them (Fig. 3–2B) from the fully-grown trophozoite. The period taken for a newly invaded merozoite to grow and differentiate into a ripe or mature gametocyte which will undergo gametogenesis, i.e. produce gametes, if taken up by a feeding mosquito, is usually 6–12 hours longer than the asexual cycle.

3.2.3   Stages in the mosquito 7

There are two types of gametocytes: female or macrogametocytes and male or microgametocytes. There is no nuclear reorganization or division within the gametocytes while they are in the vertebrate host. If, however the mature gametocytes are taken in the blood meal into the mid-gut of the vector, they lose the red cell membrane and undergo gametogenesis.

Within about 10 minutes the microgametocyte divides mitotically three times to give 8 nuclei which migrate into 8 flagella (Fig. 3–2b) which extrude and then detach. These flagella are the microgametes which swim speedily through the blood meal.

Meanwhile, the macrogametocyte on shedding the red cell membrane has become the macrogamete and is now primed for fertilization.

Fertilization occurs within a few minutes of the release of the microgametes and the nuclei fuse forming a zygote. Over the next 12–18 hours the spherical zygote transforms into the oval leaf-shaped ookinete, 7–18 μm in length and 2.5 μm in diameter. The ookinete is equipped with the same organelles as the other invasive stages: apical complex, mitochondria, microtubules, nucleus and is covered by two membranes. Within 24 hours the mature ookinete crosses the gut wall, usually passing intracellularly through the mid-gut epithelium, and eventually comes to rest extracellularly between the basement cell membrane and the basal lamina of the mid-gut wall of the mosquito. There the parasite rounds up and redifferentiates into an oocyst, losing the apical complex and microtubules. Over the next 10–12 days the oocyst is seen to grow, its diameter increasing from about 10 to over 50 μm. After 2 to 4 days a capsule or oocyst wall is formed. The oocyst has no cytostome, presumably taking its nutrients in through the surface. The point in the life cycle of malaria parasites at which meiosis occurs is not known (see Chapter 6) but it is probably in the zygote soon after fertilization, the nuclear divisions which occur during the first 7 days in the oocyst after this being mitotic. By day 7 numerous nuclei are present in the oocyst cytoplasm forming a syncytium known as the sporoblastoid body. Sporozoite buds now form on the outer membrane of the sporoblastoid body. Within each bud polar rings, micronemes and microtubules differentiate and endoplasmic reticulum, ribosomes and mitochondria migrate into the emerging sporozoite. The nuclei undergo a final division and a single nucleus enters each sporozoite which detaches from the sporoblastoid body to lie free in the oocyst capsule. Several thousands of sporozoites are produced within each oocyst and a single mosquito may carry several hundred oocysts on its mid-gut. The sporozoites are finally released from the oocyst into th‾ haemocoel of the vector, either through the capsule wall rupturing, or possibly through small holes in the capsule wall. Via the haemocoel the sporozoites reach and penetrate into the lumen of the salivary glands. The sporozoites may remain viable for an indefinite period until discharge during frequent blood meals. The time taken for malaria parasites to complete the cycle (sporogony) in the vector depends upon the external environmental conditions, particularly those of temperature and humidity, with maximum and minimum temperatures for each species of malaria above and below which the parasites fail to thrive. For example, *P. vivax* can complete sporogony at temperatures between 16°C and 30°C, whereas *P. falciparum* requires a minimum of 18°C. Sporogony in *P. vivax* can be completed in 9 days at 24–25°C and 16 days at 20°C.

3.3   Avian malarias

Birds and reptiles differ from mammals in one major way and that is in the site of the exo-erythrocytic development of the malaria parasite. In birds this takes place in the fixed tissue cells of the reticulo-endothelial system rather than the liver. In addition there are cycles of secondary exo-erythrotic schizogony with the tissue cells being invaded by merozoites coming from exo-erythrocytic and even erythrocytic schizonts. In one of the most common avian malarias, *P. relictum*, there are at least three cycles of exo-erythrocytic multiplication which are referred to, in order of their development as cryptozoites, metacryptozoites and phanerozoites and the tissues invaded include the lungs, brain and spleen.

3.4   Circadian rhythms and transmission

A striking feature of the asexual cycle in the erythrocytes of mammalian malarias is that the parasites tend to grow in synchrony with one another and the length of the asexual cycle is 24 hours or multiples of 24 hours: the parasite has a very accurate biological clock. Does this clock benefit the parasite in any way? Working with *P. knowlesi* and *P. cynomolgi* in monkeys and *P. cathemerium* in canaries, Hawking and his colleagues put forward the hypothesis that the regular asexual cycle is connected with the transmission of the parasite by night-biting mosquitoes. They conclude from their experiments that ripe gametocytes are not long-lived and have a peak of infectivity for the mosquito during the middle of the night. Ripe gametocytes in the blood are most infective therefore around the time of peak mosquito activity, thereby facilitating transmission. The development of ripe gametocytes from merozoites released from schizont-infected red cells takes a defined period, usually a few hours longer than the asexual cycle. The synchronous asexual cycle ensures that new merozoites are produced at about the same time each day, and that therefore the gametocytes which develop from them will also reach maturity at about the same time each night when the mosquitoes feed. The timing of the asexual cycle appears to be governed by the cycle of body temperature. In monkeys, which were artificially cooled during the day and warmed during the night, erythrocytic schizogony was switched from midday to midnight.

3.5   Malaria parasites of man

3.5.1   Plasmodium falciparum–*malignant tertian malaria*

This most deadly of the human malarias, is confined to the tropics and subtropics. In Africa it is responsible for more deaths than any other single cause. The pre-erythrocytic cycle lasts 5½ days, each liver schizont releasing about 30 000 merozoites. During the last 12 hours of the 48-hour asexual erythrocytic cycle the parasitized red cells sequester in capillaries of internal organs, attaching through 'knobs' on the red cell. The crescent-shaped gametocytes are mature in 10–12 days. Most patients surviving the acute phase of the infection, when 25% or more of red cells may be infected, remain infected for 7–9 months.

3.5.2   Plasmodium vivax–*benign tertian malaria*

Although once common in temperate countries, such as southern England, *P. vivax* is now found only in the subtropics. The pre-erythrocytic cycle lasts 8 days, each schizont producing about 10 000 merozoites. Some sporozoites on entering the liver become dormant, as hypnozoites, which resume their development months later to cause true relapses. Merozoites preferentially invade young red cells with parasitaemias rarely exceeding 1%. The asexual erthrocytic cycle last 48 hours. Gametocytes take 4 days to become infective to the mosquito. Relaspes in *P. vivax* infections are common.

3.5.3   Plasmodium malariae–*quartan malaria*

Eradicated from temperate countries *P. malariae* is now relatively uncommon. The pre-erythrocytic cycle takes 15 days, each mature liver schizont containing approximately 15 000 merozoites. Merozoites are said to prefer mature red cells although parasitaemias usually remain less than 1%. In red cells the asexual cycle is complete in 72 hours. After the primary attack the infection becomes chronic and can persist for more than 50 years.

3.5.4   Plasmodium ovale

P. ovale is rare, most cases occurring in West Africa. The liver cycle lasts 9 days and each liver schizont produces about 15 000 merozoites. The asexual erythrocytic cycle takes about 48 hours. The patent parasitaemias always remain low. In blood smears the infected cells are oval rather than round and hence the specific name *ovale*.

3.6 Some malaria parasites of animals which are used in the laboratory

3.6.1 Non-human primate malarias

The malaria parasites of non-human primates are very similar to those infecting man and indeed some of them are separated from human parasites only with difficulty. Some 20 species are now recognized. The similarity between human and non-human primate malarias make the latter good laboratory models of human malaria providing suitable laboratory hosts are available. *P. knowlesi* and *P. cynomolgi* are referred to in this book.

P. knowlesi is common in kra and long-tailed macaques in Malayan jungles. In the natural host the infection takes a mild course of long duration. Nearly all laboratory investigations with this parasite have employed the rhesus monkey, *Macaca mulatta*, which until recently was imported into Europe and the U.S.A. in large numbers from India and Pakistan. In the rhesus the hitherto benign *P. knowlesi* becomes a lethal parasite killing the host with a fulminating parasitaemia within about 2 weeks of sporozoite infection. The asexual erythrocytic cycle takes 24 hours. *P. cynomolgi* is found in various kra monkeys in India and S.E. Asia. In the laboratory it is usually kept in rhesus monkeys. It has a 48-hour asexual erythrocytic cycle.

3.6.2 Rodent malarias

Up to the late 1940s screening of compounds for anti-malarial activity was mainly carried out using avian malarias in canaries, chickens and ducks, and to a lesser extent using simian malarias. In 1948 malaria parasites were discovered in small rodents, thicket rats, in the Congo (now Zaire) and these parasites were found to be infective to mice and rats. A malaria parasite thus became available which would infect the cheapest and most easily maintained laboratory animal, the mouse. The complete life cycle of this parasite, named *P. berghei* after a Belgian malariologist was not fully described until 17 years later by Yoeli and Most. By that time, 1965, over 500 scientific articles had been written describing work with *P. berghei* which gives a measure of the significance of the discovery of this parasite.

Since the middle 1960s further rodent malaria parasites have been isolated in West and Central Africa and adapted to laboratory rodents. The taxonomy of these rodent parasites has been difficult to sort out. Four species of rodent malarias are now recogized – *P. berghei, P. yoelii, P. vinckei* and *P. chabaudi*. The latter three species each contain two or more sub-species.

3.6.3 Avian malarias

In the middle 1920s *P. cathemerium* from the American house sparrow and *P. relictum* from a variety of passerines were found to infect canaries and these two species provided the basis of experimental work on avian malarias, including the screening of compounds for anti-malarial activity. Canaries were expensive laboratory hosts, however, and it was therefore an important landmark when *P. gallinaceum*, the natural parasite of the jungle fowl in Asia and the Far East, and *P. lophurae* were found to infect the inexpensive domestic chickens and ducks respectively. *P. gallinaceum*, in particular, was the avian malaria used for drug-screening until the rodent malarias superseded them.

4 Pathology and Diagnosis

4.1 Pathology of human malaria

In discussing the clinical symptoms of malaria we will use *P. falciparum* as our example because this is the most pathogenic of human malarias. The incubation period, i.e. the interval between the infective bite and the patient becoming unwell, is 8 to 14 days. The first symptoms are very similar to those of influenza or a hangover – headache, fever, general body pain and gastrointestinal upsets. It is the parasites in the blood which cause the illness. *P. falciparum* has a 48-hour asexual cycle (see Chapter 3) in the blood and correspondingly in many patients a regular tertian fever may occur. Fever is associated with the bursting of the schizont-infected red cells. In other patients, however, fevers are irregular. The feverish period usually lasts less than a half a day, and is characterized by a high temperature, when the patient feels cold and shivers, and a hot phase when the patient sweats. In between fevers the patient can feel quite well. What actually causes the high temperature is not properly understood but it is thought that some substance(s), possibly derived from the parasite itself, stimulate the release of a pyrogen (fever inducing substance) from white cells. The pyrogen precipitates a sequence of events in the brain which results in a restricted blood flow in the peripheral capillaries and a consequent failure to dissipate heat which in turn causes the body temperature to rise. In *P. malariae* and *P. vivax* infections the fevers tend to show a 72 hour and 48 hour periodicity respectively (Fig. 4–1).

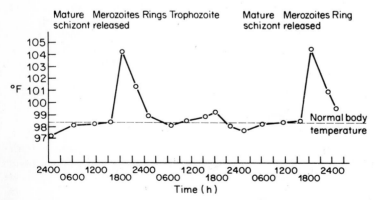

Fig. 4–1 Temperature chart of a patient with a *P. vivax* infection. Note how schizogony (every 48 hours) just precedes a rise in temperature.

If the number of *P. falciparum* parasites increases in the blood unchecked by natural or acquired resistance or anti-malarial drugs, the patient's condition will become serious and he may die. The severity of the disease is usually proportional to the number of parasitized red cells. The effect of the parasite on the normal structure and functioning of the patient's body are numerous and complex. The most obvious effect is that on the red cells. Red cells are directly destroyed by the parasite. Parasitized and non-parasitized red cells are phagocytosed by the body's phagocytic cells, particularly in the liver and spleen. It is not clear why some non-infected red cells are removed before their normal life span is completed. Possibly auto-immune reactions, i.e. immune responses to the body's own constituents, are induced including reactions to certain red cells, as a result of which the latter are prematurely destroyed. Loss of red cells means anaemia. As *P. falciparum* reaches the late trophozoite stage the parasitized red cell becomes more adhesive to the endothelial lining of capillaries and sinusoids of the internal organs. The capillaries become congested with parasitized red cells, and can become blocked preventing the normal flow of blood. The consequences of this are serious. First the blocked vessels may burst as pressure builds causing haemorrhages: the loss of blood into the tissues contributes further to anaemia. In the brain, blockage of blood vessels causes convulsions and cerebral malaria in which there are numerous signs of nervous disorder and eventually coma.

Anaemia and occlusion of capillaries together may starve the organs and tissues of oxygen and anoxia ensues which damages the affected area. If the destruction of red cells is intense, free haemoglobin is liberated into the plasma and this is then excreted in the urine, a condition known as haemoglobinuria. In blackwater fever, a now rare complication of *P. falciparum* malaria, there is rapid intravascular haemolysis. This is associated with irregular drug treatment, particularly of quinine.

Post mortem examination of fatal cases of *P. falciparum* reveals damage to kidneys, liver, lungs and the brain. Haemorrhages around the blocked blood vessels in the brain are seen. The spleen and liver are enlarged and discoloured because their phagocytic cells have taken up malarial pigment.

Although infections with the other human malarias can be unpleasant they are rarely fatal. The patient will have fevers, feel unwell and perhaps become anaemic. (Tropical splenomegaly and the nephrotic syndrome associated with malaria are discussed in Chapter 8.)

4.2   Diagnosis of human malaria

A definite diagnosis of malaria depends on finding parasites in the blood. This is because the symptoms of malaria, particularly fever, are shared with numerous other ailments. A wrong diagnosis in the case of a *P. falciparum* infection may result in an unnecessary fatality. The parasites in the blood are detected by making on a slide thick and thin blood smears from a finger prick, staining the smears with Field's or Giemsa's stain, and then searching the smear under the high power of the microscope. The thick smears permit examination of a greater number of red cells. The thin smear is useful for identifying the species of the parasite. In the case of *P. falciparum* it may be necessary to take blood smears on several occasions during 48 hours to be sure that smears are taken when the ring stage parasites are circulating in the peripheral blood.

5 Biochemistry

Details of the biochemistry of the malaria parasite, apart from their intrinsic interest, are of particular importance in the search for new anti-malarials and in understanding the mode of action of existing drugs. The points where host and parasite differ in some aspect of their biochemical processes may provide the targets for anti-malarial substances (see Chapter 9). Unfortunately our knowledge of the biochemistry of malaria parasites, although accumulating, is still relatively scanty and what is known mainly pertains to the intra-erythrocytic asexual stages. It is not difficult to see why this is. The technical problems are considerable and as one author put it, 'Biochemical investigations on *Plasmodium* are not for the faint of heart'. The major difficulty is that of obtaining viable parasites, which may need to be free of host materials, a difficult task even for some extracellular parasitic protozoa and more so for an intracellular parasite. The most readily available stage of *Plasmodium* for most species is the intra-erythrocytic asexual stage, which is usually obtained by bleeding a heavily infected host. Continuous *in vitro* culture may provide the same material but this is possible at present with a very few species. Removing the parasite from the red cell is difficult. Before a metabolic or enzymic process can be safely said to occur within the erythrocytic parasite it must be certain that this process is not due to contaminating plasma, white blood cells, platelets or red cells. The following is a summary of what is known about the basic biochemistry of plasmodia and unless otherwise indicated refers to the intra-erythrocytic stages.

5.1 Carbohydrates and energy production

Plasmodia require energy for various processes such as biosyntheses, reproduction and locomotion (in some stages). Mammals utilize glycogen and lipid as their major energy store. Malaria parasites do not store glycogen or any other polysaccharide although the avian malarias may use lipid as an energy store. Glucose, abundant in the host's blood, appears to be the main energy substrate. In order to reach the parasite glucose must pass through the red cell membrane and the membranes of the parasitophorous vacuole. This readily occurs and is a process which consumes little energy. This is because the presence of the parasite in the red cell has the effect of increasing the permeability of the red cell membrane to glucose and many more complex molecules. That is, the red cell loses some of its regulatory powers over the passage of molecules across the red cell membrane. In mammalian malarias glucose catabolism is via glycolysis, most of the glucose being converted to lactate: in these parasites the mitochondria are acristate and lack the tricarboxylic acid (TCA) cycle for the further catabolism of pyruvate.

Although the parasites lack the TCA cycle there is evidence that they have a cytochrome-containing electron transport chain with oxygen as the terminal acceptor but there is no evidence yet that this is coupled to energy production. Cytochrome oxidase has been reported, but no other cytochromes. It could be that this enzyme is not involved in a respiratory process but in the biosynthesis of nucleic acids. The bird malarias, in contrast to the mammalian malarias, do have cristate mitochondria and a functional TCA cycle. Some glucose may, in this case, be metabolized beyond pyruvate to carbon dioxide and water. In mammals the phosphoglucanate pathway, although energy-yielding, has other functions, one of which is the conversion of hexoses to pentoses which are required for nucleic acid synthesis. A partial phosphogluconate pathway is present in *Plasmodium* for the provision of pentoses. Histochemical studies on the biochemistry of carbohydrates in stages other than the intra-erythrocytic stages suggest that the mature gametocytes, oocysts, and sporozoites of *P. berghei* have cristate mitochondria, some of the TCA cycle and electron transport chain.

5.2   Nucleic acids

Nucleic acids are made up of purine and pyrimidine nucleotides. In mammals purines are both synthesized *de novo* and obtained by salvage pathways. Malaria parasites, in common with many other parasitic protozoa, are incapable of synthesizing purines *de novo* and are dependent on salvage pathways. Hypoxanthine appears to be the preferred purine and is derived from the catabolism of ATP of the red cell. Pyrimidines are synthesized *de novo* in mammals and also in plasmodia. That plasmodia synthesize pyrimidines *de novo* complements the *in vitro* observations that pyrimidines are transported into the red cells very slowly.

Malaria parasites contain DNA and RNA. The DNA is thought to be double stranded and linear and the base composition (guanine plus cytosine or G + C content) is characteristic for each group of plasmodia. RNA is present as ribosomal, transfer and, it is assumed, messenger RNA, the ribosomal RNA having a base composition similar to other protozoa.

5.3   Protein metabolism

Mammals use twenty amino acids in the synthesis of their protein components of which ten, the so-called essential amino acids, must be taken up in the diet. Mammals can synthesize the remaining ten amino acids from the essential amino acids. Malaria parasites also utilize the twenty amino acids but it is not known how many must be acquired preformed. For the parasites the amino acids come from three sources: (*i*) biosynthesis within the parasite; (*ii*) uptake of free amino acids from the plasma or the host cell and (*iii*) by the enzymatic breakdown of host cell haemoglobin by parasite proteinases. The degradation of haemoglobin is incomplete, leaving the residue as malarial pigment or haemozoin. The exact composition and function of the pigment is unknown. Protein synthesis in malaria parasites is thought to be similar to that in mammals. A well-characterized protein from *P. lophurae* is the histidine-rich protein (HRP). This protein has a molecular weight of 35–40 000 daltons and as the name implies is particularly rich in histidine residues. It is found in granules in the cytoplasm of trophozoites and possibly in the polar organelles of merozoites and because of this latter location it may be involved in the invasion of red cells by merozoites by causing extension and invagination of cell membranes.

5.4 Folate metabolism

Tetrahydrofolate (THF) is important in the interconversion of certain amino acids, and the synthesis of purine nucleotides, among other functions. Malaria parasites synthesize THF *de novo* from para-amino benzoic acid, glutamate and guanosine triphosphate. An intermediate on this pathway is dihydrofolate which is then converted to THF, the reaction being catalyzed by the enzyme dihydrofolate reductase. The importance of dihydrofolate reductase as a target for the 'antifol' anti-malarial drugs, such as pyrimethamine, and the sulphonamides is described in Chapter 9.

As noted in the Introduction one aim of the biochemist attempting to unravel the biochemistry of the malaria parasite is to reveal differences in the metabolic processes of the parasite and host in the hope that these differences can be exploited in the development of anti-malarial drugs. Differences have been demonstrated, some of which are noted above, but with few exceptions these differences have not yet been exploited. Investigation of the biochemistry of plasmodia will no doubt become more fruitful as biochemical and parasito-logical procedures improve and, in due course, further potential targets for anti-malarials will come to light. Today's biochemist is, perhaps, more aware than his predecessors of the difficulties and the potential pitfalls to be encountered when working with malaria parasites and for this reason progress may be more rapid and more certain, and, it is hoped, will embrace all stages of the malaria parasites.

6 Genetics of Malaria Parasites

In 1921 it was reported that the avian malaria parasite, *P. relictum* , could develop resistance to the anti-malarial quinine. Since that time drug-resistance to many anti-malarials has been described in experimental and human malarias (see Chapter 9). Thus within the same species of malaria parasite there are populations which differ in repect of at least one stable characteristic, i.e. drug sensitivity. Such was our understanding of the genetics of malaria parasites at the time when drug-resistance to human malaria parasites was first described, some 25 years ago, that it was possible only to speculate on if, and how, factors such as drug-resistance might spread through the populations of malaria parasites. Techniques have now been developed which permit the kind of genetic analyses, which have been routine with some free-living protozoa, to be carried out on malaria parasites. Our present knowledge of the genetics of malaria parasites come mainly from work on rodent malaria parasites by Beale, Walliker and colleagues in Edinburgh.

Malaria parasites have sexual stages which give rise to gametes in the gut of the mosquito. The factor(s) which determine the sex of a gametocyte are unknown but it is thought that gametocytogenesis is controlled by physiological mechanisms rather than by genetic control. The evidence for this conclusion comes from the facts that (*i*) populations of erythrocytic parasites derived from a single parasitized red cell, i.e. clones, still produce both male and female gametocytes and (*ii*) all the stages seen in erythrocytes are almost certainly derived from a haploid stage (see below). These two facts are not compatible with the idea that segregation of sex chromosomes or of genes which determine sex, is responsible for gametocyte formation.

Fertilization in the mid-gut of the mosquito results in the formation of a diploid zygote. As the blood stage parasites, both asexual and sexual, are almost certainly haploid, there must be a meiotic or reduction division in the interval between zygote formation and the prodution of the erythrocytic stages in the next host. This division could occur in the mosquito or during pre-erythrocytic schizogony in the liver. The latter is thought to be a remote possibility and it is assumed that meiosis of a kind occurs during one of the divisions which immediately follow fertilization. One of the problems which make it difficult to pinpoint meiosis is that the nuclear chromatin in *Plasmodium* does not condense in the normal way so that the chromosomes have never been seen as distinct structures by light or electron microscopy. That chromosomes exist is deduced from ultrastructural observations, which show the presence of structures called kinetochores, in malaria parasites. These are thought to play a part in arranging the chromosomes on the spindle tubules and in the subsequent segregation of the genetic material during cell division. The cytological data suggest that the haploid chromosome number is 8 to 10. In the Coccidia, which are protozoan parasites related to malaria parasites, meiosis is unusual in that it is a one-step division and no chiasmata are formed between chromosomes. Should this form of reduction division occur in *Plasmodium* then crossing-over would not be expected and genetic recombination would be restricted to chromosome reassortment.

Before genetic analysis of an organism can be attempted, a number of criteria need to be satisfied. It must be possible to carry out controlled matings between defined strains or lines of that organism, and these strains or lines must have suitable stable characters which can be used as genetic markers in these crosses. It must also be possible to clone the organism, i.e. to derive populations from a single organism. At the present time genetic studies on *Plasmodium* mainly depend on the use of laboratory animals. The procedures employed in cloning malaria parasites involve micromanipulation or a dilution method. In the former method individual parasitized red cells are picked out of a suspension of red cells under the microscope and injected into recipient animals. In the dilution method infected blood is diluted until, for example, there is on average about one parasite in 1 ml of diluent and each recipient animal is given 0.1 ml of diluent intravenously. It can be calculated that statistically 96% of the infections which subsequently develop in the recipients are clones. Whatever the method of cloning, in practice large numbers of experimental animals are required. The rodent plasmodia are a particularly good choice for genetical studies because (*i*) there are now four species, and numerous strains of each species, available, most of them isolated in the field, (*ii*) they can be mosquito transmitted, and (*iii*) the experimental hosts, mice, are relatively inexpensive and readily available.

The genetic markers utilized in rodent malarias are enzyme polymorphism (see below), drug-resistance, strain-specific cross-immunity, virulence and to a lesser extent host specificity. Enzyme polymorphism and differences relating to antigenic structure (which determine the degree of cross-immunity between strains) are naturally occurring differences, whereas drug resistance and virulence are produced by induction and/or selection in the laboratory.

Using the technique of electrophoresis the proteins in the soluble extracts of malaria parasite migrate at different rates, and after a set time reach positions in the starch gel which are determined mainly by the overall charge of each protein. Enzymes in the extracts can be subsequently identified and located in the gel by applying stains specific for particular enzymes. Different electrophoretic forms of the same enzyme can therefore be distinguished by the position they occupy after electrophoresis for a fixed time under defined conditions. Enzymes are polypeptides and since polypeptides are directly related to genes, i.e. are the products of single genetic loci, variations in the eletrophoretic form of an enzyme reflect gene differences and thus can be used as a genetic markers. Blood stage parasites are released from their red cell using a detergent, saponin, and then lysed by freezing and thawing in water several times. The soluble proteins are collected by removing the insoluble material by centrifugation. Four enzymes have been most frequently studied:

glucose phosphate isomerase (GPI), 6-phosphogluconate dehydrogenase (6PGD), lactate dehydrogenase (LDH), and NADP-dependent glutamate dehydrogenase. Several variants of each of the four enzymes have been identified for *P. berghei, P. yoelii, P. chabaudi* and *P. vinckei*, and each species of *Plasmodium* has its own characteristic enzymes forms. Enzyme variation has also been detected in *P. falciparum* but no genetical studies can be carried out on this parasite at the present time. Each electrophoretic form of an enzyme is given a code number.

Drug resistance as a genetic marker has been mainly restricted to the resistance of asexual blood stages to the anti-malarials pyrimethamine and chloroquine, and is recognized as a feature of a population of parasites when the parasites continue to grow in the presence of the drug given at a dose rate which eliminates drug-sensitive parasites. In the laboratory drug-insensitive 'lines' can be produced by exposing the parasites to a steadily increasing level of drug. Such resistant lines may be very stable: for example, a cloned pyrimethamine resistant line of *P. yoelii* remained stable after 55 blood passages, 18 mosquito transmissions and 5 months' storage in liquid nitrogen.

Variation in the virulence (i.e. the rate at which the primary parasitaemias increase and/or the proportion of infected hosts which die) of different strains of *Plasmodium* species, particularly the rodent plasmodia, is well known. Although the virulence of a parasite may be influenced by non-genetic factors such as the age of the host, the host's diet, and the presence of other infecting organisms, it is now established that genetic factors also play a part.

The typical format of the experiments which the Edinburgh group carried out to demonstrate that genetic recombination occurs in malaria parasites is as follows: Mixtures were made of blood containing equal proportions of gametocytes of two cloned lines (a line is a parasite population which is passaged from one host to another) of parasites which differed with respect to at least two pairs of genetic markers. Mosquitoes were fed on the mixed bloods and gametes produced. As cross- and self-fertilization should occur statistically with equal frequency, the resulting zygotes should theoretically consist of 50% hybrids and 25% of each parental line (see below and Fig. 6–1). In the hybrid zygotes recombination should occur at meiosis. The zygotes completed development to give sporozoites which were used to infect mice. Infection of the blood eventually occurred, clones were prepared and their genetic markers categorized. If cross-fertilization had occurred recombinants would be found. Control infections were set up to ensure that spontaneous mutation did not occur in the parental lines and also that recombination only occurred after cross-fertilization and not simply by mixing of the two lines.

The following experiment with *P. chabaudi* carried out by Walliker and colleagues used such a procedure. Crosses were made with two lines of *P. chabaudi* which differed with respect to two enzyme markers and sensitivity to pyrimethamine. The two parental lines were 411AS, which was pyrimethamine resistant and had enzyme forms 6PGD–2 and LDH–3, and 96AJ characterized by pyrimethamine sensitivity and enzymes 6PGD–3 and LDH–2. Seventy clones were subsequently prepared from the progeny of the cross of which 15

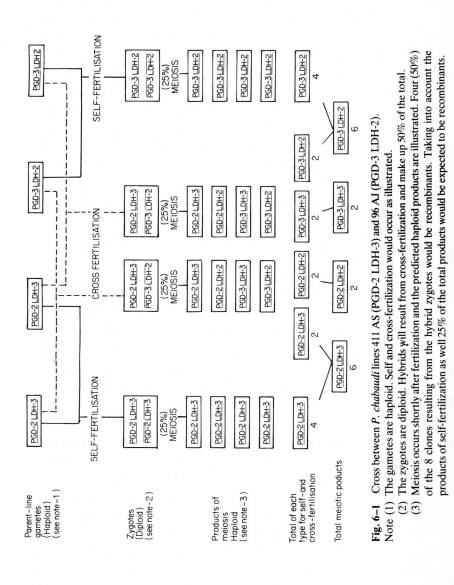

Fig. 6-1 Cross between *P. chabaudi* lines 411 AS (PGD-2 LDH-3) and 96 AJ (PGD-3 LDH-2).

Note (1) The gametes are haploid. Self and cross-fertilization would occur as illustrated.

(2) The zygotes are diploid. Hybrids will result from cross-fertilization and make up 50% of the total.

(3) Meiosis occurs shortly after fertilization and the predicted haploid products are illustrated. Four (50%) of the 8 clones resulting from the hybrid zygotes would be recombinants. Taking into account the products of self-fertilization as well 25% of the total products would be expected to be recombinants.

were recombinants for the enzyme markers. If it is assumed that self- and cross-fertilization occurs with equal frequency it would be expected that 50% (i.e. 35) of the zygotes would be hybrids (Fig. 6–1). If the genes controlling the two enzymes are independently assorted, half of the clones (i.e. 17.5) coming from hybrid zygotes would theoretically be recombinant clones. As noted above 15 of the clones were recombinants for the enzyme markers which is very close to the theoretical figure of 17.5. Examination of the clones for sensitivity to pyrimethamine revealed that the pyrimethamine-resistance character segregated independently of either enzyme marker which suggests that the two enzyme markers and pyrimethamine resistance are not linked. Further experiments showed that the other two genetic markers available, differences in virulence and differences in the antigens which are involved in the induction of anti-malarial immunity, are, like the enzyme markers and drug resistance, inherited in a Mendelian fashion.

Given that genetic recombination within the same species of *Plasmodium* can be shown to occur in the laboratory, what is the evidence that genetic mixing takes place in the wild and what are the immediate consequences of this? First, it is necessary to note that in the wild, individual thicket rats have been found infected with different species of rodent plasmodia and/or with different clones of the same sub-species and these infections are long lasting. Thus the artifical mixing of gametocytes in the laboratory also occurs naturally in the wild. Although the number of wild isolates of the different rodent plasmodia available is relativly small, there is some evidence of random matings occurring, with its consequent genetic mixing. For example, in *P. chabaudi chabaudi* there are three forms of the enzyme 6PGD and four of LDH. Assuming that random mating takes place and the various alleles are found with equal frequency 12 recombinant types should be identified with equal frequency. Twenty isolates of *P. c. chabaudi* from the Central African Republic were categorized according to their 6PGD and LDH type. Of the 12 possible enzyme combinations 9 were represented in the 20 isolates.

It is reasonable and expedient to assume that genetic mixing is a feature of all plasmodia including the human malarias. Certainly the genetic markers of enzyme variants, drug resistance and antigenic differences are well recognized in *P. falciparum*. The adaptability in the face of adverse circumstances which genetic variability confers on a parasite is of particular importance to the control of human malarias by the use of anti-malarial drugs and in due course by the use of anti-malarial vaccines. Drug resistance in the rodent plasmodia has been shown to be the result of gene mutations. Once drug resistance has appeared in human malaria it may extend through the parasite population, the limit of this spread being determined by the movements of the vector and the host. Air travel by itself has considerably widened the scope of dissemination of genes conferring drug resistance. One unexpected and alarming finding is that in the rodent parasites clones of parasites which were resistant to the anti-malarial chloroquine had an advantage over clones of drug-sensitive parasites when the two clones were grown in the same animal at the same time.

Chloroquine resistant strains of *P. falciparum* are already recognized and causing problems in South East Asia, South America and more recently there have been early signs of chloroquine resistance in Africa. If the superior vitality of the chloroquine-resistance rodent parasites is also a feature of chloroquine-resistant human malarias then chloroquine resistance may, as Walliker suggests, spread rapidly with serious consequences.

7 Natural Resistance

An animal or person surviving the acute phase of a malaria infection develops an acquired immunity which suppresses the erythrocytic infection. During the vulnerable period between the invasion of the red cells and an effective acquired immune response being mounted (see Chapter 8), some individuals have the benefit of protective mechanisms which are not part of the body's general defence system and which serve to moderate the severity of infection. Some of these protective mechanisms are genetically controlled while others may simply be incidental and reflect changing environmental factors such as the availability of food. In this chapter we shall consider how a malaria infection may be moderated by non-immune mechanisms and in addition review some of the circumstances in which, in contrast, a malaria infection may be exacerbated.

7.1 Haemoglobins and resistance to malaria

The growth of malaria parasites in the red cells is dependent on the catabolism of the haemoglobin in the red cell.

7.1.1 Sickle haemoglobin (HbS)

Sickle haemoglobin results from a mutation in the gene locus controlling the synthesis of the beta-polypeptide chain of adult haemoglobin (HbA). The result is that in each of the two mutant chains a single amino-acid substitution takes place, namely valine for glutamic acid. In individuals who are heterozygous for the sickle gene (genotype HbAS) about half the haemoglobin is HbS and the rest mainly HbA. Homozygotes for HbS (genotype HbSS) have 80% or more of their haemoglobin as HbS and the rest is mainly foetal haemoglobin (HbF). Heterozygotes are referred to as having the sickle-cell trait. The majority of children homozygous for the sickle gene die during childhood, usually from sickle-cell anaemia and therefore do not reach reproductive age. Sickle-cell heterozygotes in contrast are unlikely to suffer any obvious disability unless they are subjected to low partial pressures of oxygen, for example at high altitude, when the red cells are distorted into the sickle shape. Homozygotes show sickling at higher partial pressures of oxygen than heterozygotes. Thus we have a gene which is rarely passed on to the next generation by individuals homozygous for the gene but in much of tropical Africa, and in parts of Europe and Asia 1% of the population may be HbSS and 20–40% of the population may be HbAS. It is most unlikely that the mutation rate at the locus controlling the polypeptide of the haemoglobin molecule could account for the persistent high rate of the sickle gene. A survey in Kano State of northern Nigeria, a hyper-endemic area for *P. falciparum* , found that in 534 newborn children 24% were HbAS and in a sample of children 5–9 years old 29% were HbAS. These figures illustrate the usually high incidence of the sickle cell trait in an African population and the increase from 24 to 29% from 0 to 5 years of age suggests a survival advantage associated with it. This survival advantage is a relative protection against *P. falciparum* and hence the high frequency of the sickle gene in areas where *P. falciparum* malaria is (or was) common. In the Kano study the density and frequency of *P. falciparum* in infants up to 75 weeks of age was determined. Between the ages of 30 and 59 weeks, that is before acquired immunity had developed and after maternal passively transferred immunity had waned, the HbAS infants had a significantly lower density and frequency of *P. falciparum* asexual forms in the blood than in the infants with normal haemoglobin (genotype HbAA). Where the sickle gene is no longer put under the selective pressure of malaria as happened to the sickle trait carriers and their descendants when the carriers were transported from West Africa to the United States, its frequency diminished.

There is, therefore, no doubt that the sickle-cell trait confers some protection against *P. falciparum*. It is less clear, however, what are the cellular mechanisms whereby HbS gives this protection. It can be suggested that the merozoites fail to invade HbAS cells, or the parasites do not grow and divide as well in the HbAS cells, or the parasitized HbAS red blood cells are more readily removed by the patient's defence system than parsitized HbAA cells.

There is no reason to believe that the single amino acid difference between normal adult and sickle haemoglobin renders the latter a less suitable food source for the parasite. An early suggestion (1954) was that *P. falciparum* caused HbAS red cells to sickle *in vivo* and that sickled cells were preferentially phagocytosed. This proposal gained some support from the observation that a parasitized red cell containing HbS is more likely to sickle *in vitro* as oxygen is lost from the red cell. Recent investigations into the protective effect of HbS have used *in vitro* cultures of *P. falciparum* in which the merozoites, on release from HbAA red cells, were allowed to invade HbAS, HbSS and HbAA red cells under normal or reduced oxygen tension and the invasion rate and growth of the parasites subsequently monitored. In some cultures *in vivo* conditions were simulated in so far as parasites were cultured to the early trophozoite stage in aerobic conditions (corresponding to the period *in vivo* when the parasites are circulating in well oxygenated peripheral blood) and for the final 12 hours of the cultures, the parasites were kept in reduced oxygen tension (correponding to the final maturation period the parasite spends in the poorly oxygenated deeper tissues such as the brain, liver and spleen). The results showed that under aerobic conditions the invasion rate into HbAA, HbAS and HbSS cells was about the same but in reduced oxygen the invasion rate was significantly depressed in HbSS cells and less so in HbAS cells. Although under aerobic conditions the presence of HbS did retard parasite growth slightly, only under low O_2 tension (5%) did HbS cause striking retardation of parasite development. To bring this about it was not necessary for the parasitized red cells to sickle. The question is how does the HbS exert its harmful effect? In HbSS cells under low oxygen tension needle-like aggregates of deoxy-haemoglobin S can be seen when examined by the electron microscope, and these aggregates disrupt the parasite. In HbAS cells mechanical disruption seems unlikely and it is suggested that a loss of intracellular potassium is the cause of death. It is still unclear whether the sickling of HbAS cells is important in reducing *P. falciparum* proliferation as it is unlikely that HbAS cells sickle *in vivo*.

The experimental evidence has shown us that both HbAS and HbSS red cells are unfavourable to *P. falciparum* under certain conditions. These observations are difficult to reconcile, however, with the reported observations that HbSS patients can suffer severe *P. falciparum* infections. Explanations for this apparent anomaly may rest with the facts that, first, HbSS patients frequently lack a spleen, an organ which is very important in the development of acquired immunity to malaria parasites, and secondly, that in HbSS patients the red cell population has more young red cells than in normal people and it is now known that *P. falciparum* has a preference for young red cells.

7.1.2   Foetal haemoglobin (HbF)

In the developing human foetus initially all the haemoglobin produced is of the foetal type (HbF). Around mid-pregnancy the production of the HbA starts. At birth HbF production ceases and at this time approximately 20% of the haemoglobin is HbA and 80% HbF. By 2 months 50% of the haemoglobin is HbA and at 4 months this has risen to about 90%. During the early weeks of life infection rates with *P. falciparum* are relatively low indicating some temporary resistance. Part of this resistance may be a consequence of passively transferred anti-parasitic antibody from the mother and because the population of red blood cells present at that time is weighted towards older red cells which are less suitable for *P. falciparum*. It is, however, possible that HbF is less suitable for the proliferation of malaria parasites. Some evidence in support of this comes from children suffering from ß-thalassemia.

In children with ß-thalassemia HbF production persists for longer than is usual during the first few years of life. Children who are homozygous for ß-thalassemia rarely surive to adulthood and reproduce. In spite of this selection pressure the high frequency of ß-thalassemia in malarious or formerly malarious areas such as Sardinia, Greece and parts of South-East Asia suggests strongly that ß-thalassemia confers some resistance to malaria, and this is responsible for the high frequency of the gene carrying it.

By culturing *P. falciparum in vitro* in the presence of red cells containing HbF it has been possible to compare the ability of the parasite to invade and grow in red cells containing HbF and in red cells containing HbA. It was found that the susceptibility to invasion did not correlate with the type of haemoglobin but that the growth of *P. falciparum* in HbF-containing red cells was retarded. Thus it is possible that HbF might confer some selective advantage on children with ß-thalassemia during infancy and early childhood, at the time that a protective immunity is developing. The mechanism by which HbF impairs parasite growth is not known.

7.1.3   Haemoglobin C (HbC)

Another haemoglobin variant of HbA is HbC. In some West African populations HbA, HbS and HbC are all found. Although it is suspected that HbC may give some protection against malaria, proof from population studies and field data on infected individuals carrying the HbC gene is not forthcoming. Homozygous genotype (HbCC) individuals suffer at worst only a mild haemolytic anaemia. In culture, however, the growth of *P. falciparum* was impaired in HbCC red cells when compared with that in HbAC and HbAA cells. Of interest was that in conditions of reduced oxygen tension *P. falciparum* proliferated less well in cultures containing HbSC cells than HbAS cells. That is, HbC increased the resistance conferred by HbS.

7.2   Red cell surface and age of the red cells

7.2.1   Red cell surface

In order to invade a red cell the merozoite must attach to the red cell surface membrane and this attachment is thought to be through specific receptor sites on the red cell surface. The specificity for a particular host species which is exhibited by malaria parasites is reflected in their interaction (*in vitro*) with red cells of the preferred and not preferred hosts. For example, *P. knowlesi* will not infect guinea-pigs and correspondingly *P. knowlesi* merozoites will not even attach to guinea-pig red cells in culture. *P. knowlesi* will infect most human erythrocytes in culture but not after the red cells have been treated with the enzymes chymotrypsin and pronase. This suggests that there are receptors for the parasite on the red cell membrane and that these receptors are protein or glycoprotein in nature. Human erythrocytes lacking the Duffy blood group antigen, however, are refractory to invasion by *P. knowlesi* although in this case the merozoites attach but cannot enter the red cell. Individuals with red cells lacking the Duffy blood group antigen (genotype FyFy) are found in high frequency in West Africa where *P. vivax* is absent. The Duffy antigen may be the receptor for attachment and invasion by *P. vivax* and hence individuals lacking it are refractory to this parasite. In an Amerian experiment 11 volunteers were exposed to the bite of *P. vivax*-infected mosquitoes. Five were refractory to the parasite and the rest became infected. Only the refractory individuals were found to be Duffy negative. Duffy negative red cells are susceptible to *P. falciparum* . The red cell receptor(s) for this parasite are not known but a sialoglycopeptide might be implicated. It is probable that the receptors on the human red cell for *P. vivax* and *P. falciparum* are different.

7.2.2   Age of red cells

The age of the red cell has an important bearing on its susceptibility to invasion by plasmodia. *P. vivax* and *P. ovale* are predominantly found in young red cells. *P. berghei* , the rodent parasite, has a preference for very young red cells, reticulocytes, and hence causes severe infections in young rats, where nearly 20% of the red cells are reticulocytes, but in adult rats, where only 4% of the red cells are reticulocytes the erythrocytic infections are mild. *P. falciparum,* in the standard textbooks, is stated to have no red cell preference, invading all ages, and consequently has no constraint placed upon it through lack of a preferred red cell type. Recent work has, however, confirmed the suggestions of some early malariologists that this malaria parasite has a preference for metabolically young red cells. This view is based on evidence from patients and from examining the ability of *P. falciparum* to invade red cells of different ages in culture. This preference for younger red cells may provide a further explanation of the low incidence of severe *P. falciparum* infections in babies. A few weeks after birth erythropoiesis virtually ceases for 2–3 months and very few young red cells are produced, thereby restricting the growth of this parasite. During the most severe *P. falciparum* infections in all ages of patients, the bone marrow can be temporarily depressed, erythropoiesis is reduced, and consequently parasite multiplication may again be constrained through lack of young red cells. Explanations for the failure of older red cells to be invaded by *P. falciparum* have included (*i*) the loss of important specific receptors on the red cell membrane as the cell matures, (*ii*) a loss of metabolic activity in the older red cells (a high metabolic rate may be important in the process of invasion) and (*iii*) older red cells are less deformable and deformation of the red cell membrane is an integral component in the invasion process.

7.3 Glucose 6-phosphate dehydrogenase deficiency

The gene controlling a deficiency of the red cell enzyme, glucose 6-phosphate dehydrogenase (G-6-PD) is sex-linked and the geographical distribution of this sex-linked mutant, in tropical Africa, Mediterranean countries, the Near East, India and parts of Asia, suggests that a deficiency in G-6-PD gives some protection against malaria. The selection pressure against G-6-PD deficiency is not strong because in the male hemizygote or the female homozygote the predisposition to suffer haemolytic anaemia occurs only under exceptional circumstances and therefore only a slight advantage with respect to malaria might be necessary to maintain the G-6-PD deficiency gene. In malarious areas individuals with *P. falciparum* malaria have been examined and ranked according to their parasitaemias and the G-6-PD content of their red cells. Interpretation of the data from this kind of study is, however, controversial. Some workers conclude that there is no clinical evidence of protection against falciparum malaria, others conclude that in the heterozygous female, at least, the gene for G-6-PD deficiency does confer some protection. If we accept the latter view an explanation is required. One suggested explanation is based on the fact that red cells which are deficient in G-6-PD are predisposed to oxidant-induced haemolysis. It has been proposed that the malaria parasite exerts an oxidant stress on the red cells and that in infected red cells deficient in G-6-PD, premature lysis would occur with the likely demise of the parasites within them.

7.4   Diet

There is little known about the effect of the host's diet or nutritional state on malaria infections. If rodents are kept on a diet of only milk, an otherwise severe malaria infection is reduced to a low level. If the milk diet is supplemented with para-amino benzoic acid (PABA) (see Chapter 5), the malaria parasites attain their normal vigour. Experiments with *P. falciparum* in the South American owl monkey *Aotus trivigatus*, have given the same result. *Aotus* on an exclusively milk diet had short-lasting instead of fulminating infections. The inhibitory effect of a PABA deficient diet is certainly operative against the erythrocytic stages and possibly the pre-erythrocytic stages as well. The inhibitory effect of an exclusively milk diet may provide us with yet another explanation of why the malaria rate in infants under one year in malarious areas is lower than is to be expected.

Diets deficient in ascorbic acid (vitamin C) and the vitamin B_6 group depressed experimental malarias. Recently it has been reported that a diet deficient in protein can depress *P. berghei* infections in rats and the authors suggest that a relationship between protein intake and parasitaemia may explain why famine relief in the Third World is sometimes accompanied by increased malaria rates.

7.5   Age of the host and susceptibility to malaria parasites

The reduced susceptibility of young babies to *P. falciparum* is referred to elsewhere (p. 31). In rats there is a dramatic decline in susceptibility to *P. berghei* after they reach 8–10 weeks. Rats apart, however, increased resistance with age does not appear to be a general phenomenon.

7.6   Pregnancy

In Africa, pregnancy, even in immune women, is accompanied by increased parasite prevalence and greater parasite densities. The reason for this is thought in part to be due to the temporary depressed state of the immune system found during pregnancy.

8 Immunology

In order to understand a brief account of the immunology of malaria some basic knowledge of the immune system and its workings is essential. The immune system in vertebrates is a complex surveillance system protecting them against invading pathogens and from cancer cells. It has a dual nature: cellular (cell-mediated) immunity mediated through lymphoid cells and humoral immunity mediated through soluble proteins in the serum. The two systems interact. The basis of this duality resides in two populations of morphologically identical lymphoid cells, called lymphocytes. These are found in the blood, tissue fluids, and in particular in the spleen and the lymph nodes. One class of lymphocytes, B cells, when activated by a pathogen differentiate into plasma cells and secrete the soluble proteins – antibodies – which can bind specifically to that pathogen. The other class of lymphocytes are known as T cells and mediate the cellular response. T cells which recognize and become activated by a pathogen can directly or indirectly lead to the elimination of the pathogen by several mechanisms (see below). The lymphocytes are all derived from the bone marrow stem cells and before they become functional must undergo a maturation process. T cells pass through the thymus to mature and hence cellular immune responses are referred to as being thymus-dependent. B cells, in the bird, mature in the bursa but in the mammal, where there is no discrete bursa, the site of B cell maturation had not been identified for certain.

In addition to lymphocytes there are other cells involved in the immune system such as monocytes, macrophages and granulocytes.

The invading organism or particle carries on it or within it substances which the host recognizes as being foreign, i.e. not part of the host. These foreign substances are called antigens and the host may, through its B cells, synthesize antibodies which bind to the antigens. For some antigens B cells need the help of certain T cells in order to synthesize the specific antibody. Antibodies belong to the class of proteins called gammaglobulins or immunoglobulins, and each antibody molecule is specific for the antigen which elicited its production. In mammals five classes of immunoglobulins are recognized in the serum. They are given the shorthand notation of IgM, IgG, IgA, IgD and IgE. On first exposure (primary response) to an antigen the mammal makes the corresponding antibody relatively slowly, peak levels being reached within about 7 days and then the levels decline. First exposure to the antigen generates immunological memory of the antigen so that further exposure to the same antigen precipitates a more rapid and vigorous antibody response (secondary response) which results in higher and longer lasting antibody levels. T-cell mediated immune responses have the same kind of kinetics following primary and secondary exposure to the antigen. Hence primary infection with a pathogen may produce clinical disease before the immune response reaches effective levels but on re-infection so rapid is the immune response that the pathogen is removed before it can achieve numbers sufficient to cause clinical symptoms. Antibodies may directly kill pathogens, sometimes in conjunction with either a group of serum proteins which are collectively known as complement, or with the help of certain lymphoid or myeloid cells (such as so-called killer or K cells). They may also promote the phagocytosis of the pathogen by macrophages.

The T cell class of lymphocytes is in fact a heterogeneous collection of slightly different kinds of T cells. We are only concerned here with the way T cells could possibly kill malaria parasites and cannot go into the complexities of T cells. After exposure and re-exposure to the pathogen, some T cells become capable of lysing and hence killing the pathogen. Others secrete a variety of polypeptides known as lymphokines which in their turn induce other cells to become active against the pathogen, e.g. macrophages may be attracted to a site and become activated thus becoming better at phagocytosing and killing the pathogen, or even killing it by direct contact. The immune mechanisms which are responsible for killing a particular pathogen are referred to as effector mechanisms.

8.1   The immune response of the vertebrate host to malaria parasites

Malaria infections can be broadly assigned to one of three categories according to the course they take. The parasite may either, (*i*) multiply and rapidly kill the host, (*ii*) be quickly controlled and eliminated from the blood of the host, or (*iii*) be reduced to low and usually sub-clinical levels after the acute phase of the infection in the blood but persist for long periods. Animals, including man which survive malaria infections and show resistance to re-infection do so because they have mounted an effective protective immune response. Where the acquired resistance is incomplete and the parasites persist, the animal is referred to as being in a state of 'premunition' and this, with respect to transmission, is better for the parasite than one in which it either rapidly kills the host or is itself rapidly eliminated. Immunity to malaria in man is acquired only after repeated exposures over several years and is mainly directed against the erythrocytic stage.

In this chapter we discuss what the protective immune mechanisms are and how they may control the parasite. Information in this area comes from observations on people living in endemic areas, individuals who are volunteers or who are deliberately infected with malaria for therapeutic reasons and from experimental animals. We must be cautious in extrapolating the results from experimental animals to man. Most attention has focused on the intra-erythrocytic asexual stage because this is the pathogenic stage. Acquired resistance to malaria parasites is usually stage and species specific and in the absence of re-infection wanes with time. Immunity to *P. falciparum*, for example, confers little protection to the other human malaria parasites.

8.1.1   Immunity to sporozoites

It has been known for many years that sporozoites which have lost their infectivity, after, for example, exposure to ultraviolet light or X-irradiation (see below), can be used to immunize protectively animals and (experimentally) man. Viable sporozoites are also now known in both animals and in man to induce a detectable antibody response. For example, in the Gambia, West Africa in 1978, more than 90% of the adult population had antibodies to sporozoites of *P. falciparum* in their blood. Less than half the children had this antibody indicating that repeated exposure to sporozoites over many years is necessary to induce its formation. It is not known whether this antibody has any protective role such as preventing the sporozoites from invading the liver parenchyma cells.

8.1.2   Immunity to the exo-erythrocytic (EE) stage

There is little known about any protective immune response to the EE stage. Antibodies which react with EE stages of *P. berghei* have been demonstrated in rats but their role, if any, in acquired resistance is not known. In rats also in which EE stages are developing or have recently completed their development, after a further injection of sporozoites the number of new EE forms which develop can be significantly less than expected. Whether this phenomenon of interference occurs in man is again unknown.

8.1.3   Immunity to the erythrocytic asexual stage

This stage of the parasite can stimulate a strong anti-malarial antibody response. Accompanying the antibody response there is an increase in the amount of immunoglobulins in the blood. The spleen is the major site of production of anti-malarial antibodies, which have a significant role in acquired resistance to the erthrocytic stage of malaria but not all anti-malarial antibodies are protective. Passive transfer of serum or the γ-globulin fraction from the serum from immune to non-immune individuals confers some protection on the recipient. For example, serum was collected from adult Gambians who were clinically immune to *P. falciparum*, and the γ-globulin fraction obtained from it was then injected into infants suffering *P. falciparum* infections. The immune γ-globulin quickly reduced the blood parasitaemia in these children.

Most of the protective activity in the serum of immune animals or man is in the IgG fraction although anti-malarial antibodies are also found in IgM and IgA classes. It is almost certain that the anti-malarial IgG contains more than one antibody with protective activity. IgG antibody is passed from mother to baby across the placenta giving the neonate some short-lasting protection. How do these antibodies work? One antibody, the so-called inhibitory antibody, at least *in vitro*, prevents merozoites free in the plasma from invading the red cells, agglutinating and then lysing them in the process. Other antibodies, opsonins, and cytophilic antibody promote the phagocytosis of parasitized red cells, particularly those containing late trophozoites and schizonts, and of free merozoites also, in the blood, liver and spleen. The early growth of the erythrocytic stages seems to proceed normally in the presence of serum antibody.

The immune response to the erythrocytic parasite is not mediated by inhibitory opsonizing and cytophilic antibody alone: it is very much more complex and the predominant immune mechanism may change as the primary infection passes from the acute to the chronic phase or after re-infection of the host. There are indications that cell-mediated mechanisms (see p. 36) play a part but precisely what part is not clear.

The synergistic anti-malarial effect of antibody and cells has been reasonably well established: opsonizing antibody promoting phagocytosis of merozoites or infected red cells by macrophages has been mentioned. The combined effect of serum which contains anti-malarial antibody and mononuclear peripheral blood cells (mainly lymphocytes) in reducing the multiplication of *P. falciparum in vitro* has recently been described. It is not known yet if these cells kill *P. falciparum in vivo* in the presence of the anti-malarial antibody. Polymorphonuclear (neutrophil) blood leucocytes will also take up and kill merozoites of *P. falciparum in vitro* .

During the declining primary parasitaemia, the morphology of erythrocytic parasites of experimental malarias frequently appears abnormal and the various forms are referred to as 'crisis' forms. It is assumed that this abnormal morphology reflects mortal injury to the parasite inflicted by the host's defence system. These crisis forms may be caused by soluble non-antibody factors which are cytotoxic to the malaria parasites and which are released into the plasma from some kind of lymphoid cell, possibly a mononuclear cell known as a natural killer cell or NK cell or macrophages.' These non-antibody factors appear to be of particular importance in controlling the primary erythrocytic parasitaemia. Later on in the infection, or after re-infection, antibody and the cell-mediated mechanisms assume predominance (Fig. 8–1).

8.2   Chronic infections and antigenic variation

Malaria infections are characteristically of long duration, the parasite surviving in the blood in spite of the host's immune response attempting to remove it; the numbers of parasites present fluctuate and occasionally produce clinical relapses. In the case of *P. vivax* infections, latent liver stages intermittently complete their development and infect the blood. In other malarias, such as *P. falciparum*, there are no latent liver stages and the persistent fluctuating blood infection must reflect either an incomplete and fluctuating immune response, for which there is some evidence, and/or the parasite somehow evading the full effects of the host's acquired resistance. The erythrocytic asexual stage of *P. knowlesi* over a period of time repeatedly changes some of the antigens (variant-antigens) presented to the host, thereby requiring the host to make a specific immune (antibody) response to each new antigenic or variant-type as it appears. This process is known as antigenic variation. By producing a new variant-type as the host's immune response

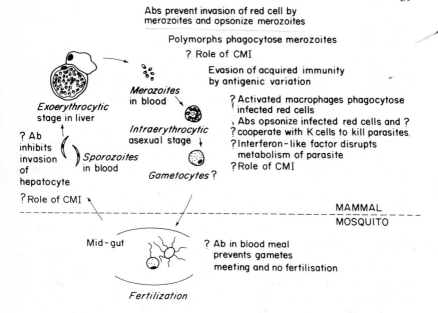

Fig. 8–1 Summary of mechanisms of acquired immunity to *Plasmodium*. Ab, antibody; ?, not known for certain; Nb, opsonizing Ab promotes phagocytosis by macrophages.

suppresses the existing variant-type, the parasite is able to keep one step ahead of the host. Usually the immune response, anti-malarial antibody being a major component of this, to each new variant as it appears is rapid and correspondingly the parasitaemia is kept low. An anti-parasitic antibody may provide the signal to the parasite to change its variant-type. The variant specific antigens in *P. knowlesi* are located in or on the red cell membrane of the schizont-infected red cell. Antigenic variation by the multiplicative blood stage is likely to be a characteristic of most or all malaria parasites but this still needs to be demonstrated. The implications of antigenic variation to the production of a vaccine against the blood stages of *Plasmodium* may be serious. Will the vaccine need to include all the possible antigenic variant types or can a vaccine be produced which transcends antigenic variation?

8.3   Vaccination

A cheap, easily administered anti-malarial vaccine would be of immense value in the control and eradication of the disease. Ideally the vaccine should consist only of those parasite antigens which induce acquired resistance and be free of contaminating host materials such as red cell antigens or adventitious agents such as viruses, and a single immunizing dose should give lasting protection to people of all ages. Such a vaccine is still a distant goal.

There are three approaches to vaccination against malaria: vaccination against sporozoites, against asexual erythrocytic stages and against sexual stages. These studies are almost entirely confined to malaria in experimental animals and the results obtained may or may not be applicable to man.

8.3.1   Immunization with sporozoites

The most successful vaccines have consisted of salivary gland sporozoites which have been attenuated, i.e. they are rendered unable to initiate an infection, by exposure to radiation such as γ-rays or X-rays. The irradiated sporozoites are most immunogenic when they are injected intravenously by syringe or through the bite of mosquitoes; the protection induced is effective against sporozoites and no other stage.

Irradiated sporozoites have been successfully used for protecting rhesus monkeys against *P. cynomolgi* and *P. knowlesi*, and, in a limited number of studies, man against *P. vivax* and *P. falciparum*: the immunity acquired was species specific.

The nature of the anti-sporozoite mechanisms (effector mechanisms) in the immunized host is not fully understood. Protection and the formation of anti-sporozoite antibody is dependent on the thymus (i.e. involves T and B cells). Antibody alone, however, does not make up the complete effector mechanism because in mice complete protection could not be given by passively transferring serum from immunized mice to naive mice and because successful sporozoite immunization was possible in mice which previously had the humoral component, but not the cell-mediated component, of their immune response depressed.

The sporozoite antigens which induce protective immunity are present on the surface membrane of salivary gland sporozoites. Anti-sporozoite antibody from an immunized host binds to these antigens, one of which is a protein, molecular weight 44 000 daltons.

It is, at present, not feasible to produce sporozoites on the scale required for commercial production of a vaccine composed of irradiated sporozoites. An alternative approach is to identify and isolate the protective sporozoite antigen(s), synthesize them using the new techniques of biotechnology and make these synthetic antigens the basis of the vaccine.

8.3.2   Immunization with asexual erythrocytic stages

It is possible to immunize experimental animals against the erythrocytic stage of rodent, simian and avian malarias and against *P. falciparum*. The vaccine has consisted of irradiated parasitized red cells, dead parasites killed by, for example, freezing and thawing or formalin, or extracts of parasites. In many cases, particularly in primates, the vaccine alone gave little protection against a challenge infection. If, however, the vaccine was given with an adjuvant such as saponin, *Bordetella pertussis* (whooping cough vaccine), or

Freund's complete adjuvant (a mixture of mineral oils containing dead *Mycobacterium butyricum*) the animals controlled a challenge infection well. An adjuvant serves to amplify the immune response to antigens. This is in contrast to the sporozoite vaccine which is effective without the assistance of an adjuvant. The effect of the erythrocytic vaccine is to reduce the level of parasitaemia and permit animals to survive an otherwise lethal infection.

One of the major hurdles to be overcome in the development of this form of vaccine is the development of procedures which enable the erythrocytic parasite to be collected free from contaminating red cell material. A vaccine containing red cell components could induce auto-immune reactions and cause haemolytic disease in the recipients. For this reason the development of methods for collecting merozoites *in vitro* after they had been released from the red cell was an exciting step forward. Merozoites of *P. chabaudi* , *P. falciparum* and, most successfully, *P. knowlesi* have been obtained. In the rhesus monkey merozoites of *P. knowlesi* incorporated in complete Freund's adjuvant injection intramuscularly give an unusually powerful resistance to challenge. Complete Freund's adjuvant cannot, however, be used in man and the search goes on for an acceptable alternative.

The gap between successful vaccination of animals and the production of a vaccine from erythrocytic stages for use in man is formidable. The difficulties of producing sufficient numbers of parasites have been lessened since Trager and Jensen in 1976 showed that *P. falciparum* could be grown continuously in red cells *in vitro* although scaling the culture method up from the small scale laboratory apparatus to the commercial will not be easy. Many workers believe that the vaccine will eventually consist of purified malarial antigens (rather than whole parasites) which had been shown to be those responsible for inducing protection, and which were synthetically produced after their compositon had been elucidated.

8.3.3 Immunization with gametocytes

Although a vaccine against the asexual erythrocytic malaria parasite would reduce the clinical disease it need not necessarily prevent transmission of the parasite. Viable gametocytes are frequently observed in the circulation of a host after the immune response has controlled the asexual erythrocytic stages. A vaccine against the male and female gametes would block fertilization in the mosquito and prevent further transmission. Chickens, rhesus monkeys and mice have been immunized against gametes of *P. gallinaceum*, *P. knowlesi* and *P. yoelii* respectively. The vaccine consisted of micro- and macrogametes and some contaminating asexual erythrocytic forms. The vaccine was usually treated with formalin or exposed to irradiation before being injected so as to render the asexual forms non-infective and an adjuvant was usually unnecessary. When the immunized animals were subsequently infected and mosquitoes allowed to feed on them, the number of oocysts developing in mosquitoes fed on the vaccinated animals was significantly less than in the mosquitoes fed on control animals, i.e. transmission was blocked. The immunity which blocked transmission was found to be mediated through anti-gamete antibodies which agglutinated the male gametes after exflagellation and thereby prevented fertilization.

8.4 Monoclonal antibodies and malaria research

In 1975, Kohler and Milstein described experiments in which they had fused mouse myeloma cells, which are tumour cells of the line which produce antibody secreting cells, and mouse spleen cells secreting antibodies to an known antigen, in their experiment sheep red cells. These fused hybrid cells are known as hybridomas and grown in culture continuously they continued to secrete the anti-sheep red cell antibody. It was found that the hybridoma cells could be cloned so that cultures could be set up in which all the hybrid cells were secreting the same antibody with defined specificity now known as a monoclonal antibody.

Using the hybridoma technique monoclonal antibodies to different stages of malaria parasite or extracts of them are now being produced. Some of these monoclonal antibodies have been found to be protective. The main reason for producing monoclonal antibodies to malarial antigens is that they provide a method for isolating purified malarial antigens, including, it is hoped, those responsible for inducing protection, and once isolated it is hoped the chemical make-up of them can be determined. Subsequently using recombinant DNA technology, it may be possible to synthesize the protective antigens in the laboratory for incorporation in a vaccine.

The analysis of the antigens of malarial parasites is not restricted to the use of monoclonal antibodies. More conventional biochemical techniques are being applied to the analysis of extracts of malaria parasites paying particular attention to membrane-bound, potentially protective, surface antigens. Antigenic chemical grouping may involve proteins, glycoproteins, glycolipids, or other complex macromolecules.

8.5   Immunosuppression

In 1962, McGregor and Barr in the Gambia immunized a group of children, who were chronically infected with *P. falciparum*, with tetanus toxoid and another group of the same age who were on anti-malarial drugs and hence were relatively free of malaria. The malarious children gave poorer antibody responses to the tetanus toxoid; the infection was causing a suppression of the children's humoral responses. Animal malarial parasites and human malaria (*P. falciparum*) are immunosuppressive, particularly during the acute patent parasitaemias and particularly with regard to thymus-dependent antibody responses. Some cell-mediated immune responses are depressed and others apparently are unaffected. How malaria exerts its immunosuppressive effect is still not clear. The implication of this immunosuppression are however important. First, children with malaria may respond poorly in vaccination programmes, for example to measles, tetanus toxoid, and other childhood vaccines. Secondly, pathogens which are normally quickly controlled and suppressed by the body's immune system when concurrent with malaria may assume unusually serious and sometimes lethal levels. It is frequently observed that malarious children develop severe bacterial infections . Thirdly, the state of immunosuppression induced by the malaria parasite may extend to the immune response by the host to the parasite itself and thereby ensure its longer survival in the host.

Burkitt's lymphoma, described by Burkitt in East Africa in 1958, is the most frequently occuring tumour in children in East Africa. Its occurrence in Africa and elsewhere in the world indicates a strong correlation between the incidence of the tumour and malaria. Malaria eradication is followed by a decrease in Burkitt's lymphoma. There is good evidence that Burkitt's lymphoma is caused by the Epstein-Barr virus (EBV). This virus in more advanced countries causes the debilitating disease glandular fever in young adults. Infection with EBV is nearly ubiquitous in African children. How malaria predisposes these children to the development of the tumour is still not clear.

8.6   Immunodiagnosis

The only sure way of diagnosing a malaria infection is by detecting parasites in blood smears. Within a few days of the erythrocytic phase becoming established, where the host survives, anti-malarial antibodies appear in the serum and various serological tests are now available for detecting these antibodies and determining the relative levels present. Demonstration of the presence of anti-malarial antibodies to the erythrocytic stages tells us that the individual has, or has had, malaria. High levels suggest a recent infection. Serological tests are rarely used for diagnosis but are very useful in epidemiological studies where the incidence and level of anti-malarial antibodies can reflect the level of transmission.

8.7   Immunopathology

Not all immune responses to malaria parasites ultimately benefit the host. Two serious conditions, tropical splenomegaly syndrome and a nephrotic syndrome, are thought in part at least to be a consequence of the immune response to malaria. Patients suffering from tropical splenomegaly syndrome (TSS) have gross and persistant enlargement of the spleen. It is found in adults in malarious areas particularly in New Guinea and West Africa, and is frequently fatal. Affected patients have high levels of anti-malarial antibodies, of IgM , of immune complexes and increased numbers of circulating B lymphocytes. The reticuloendothelial system expands to remove the immune complexes causing splenomegaly.

The nephrotic syndrome is associated with *P. malariae* and has a peak incidence in children around five years of age. Only a small proportion of cases of *P. malariae* develop the syndrome. They suffer severe renal disease manifest as oedema, oliguria (diminished amounts of urine relative to fluid intake) and proteinuria (excessive serum proteins in the urine). A biopsy of the kidneys of the unfortunate children show degeneration of the kidneys tubules and lesions on the glomeruli. The pathogenesis is thought to be related to the presence of immune complexes of soluble *P. malariae* antigen and anti-*P. malariae* antibody which circulate and become deposited in the kidney glomeruli. In a proportion of patients these complexes persist in time causing damage to glomerulus and tubule and ultimately kidney failure.

9 Chemotherapy

9.1 Anti-malarial drugs

In treating any parasitic infection with a chemotherapeutic agent the intent is that the drug will be toxic to the parasite at a concentration in the body's fluids and tissues which is not toxic to the host. It is no good killing the parasite if the host dies as well! The anti-malarial primaquine, for example, can be given at a level which kills the liver stages of the parasite but which is still toleratd by the patient. If the same drug was to be used to kill the erythrocytic stages a higher dose of the drug would be necessary but at this dose the severity of the side effects would be quite unacceptable. Hence primaquine's usefulness is only for destroying liver stages.

None of the available anti-malarial drugs are effective against all stages of the malaria parasite found in the vertebrate host. The choice of anti-malarial drug for use in man will depend on whether it is for prophylactic purposes (i.e. to prevent or to suppress clinical malaria, usually referred to as causal prophylactics) or curative purposes (i.e. to treat an acute clinical attack of malaria and/or eliminate tissue stages). It also depends on which species of malaria parasite is to be controlled. The dose of drug used will depend on its toxicity, the likely sensitivity of the parasite to that anti-malarial, the immune status, i.e. the level of acquired resistance, of the person, and whether in the long term it is of benefit to the patient to develop an effective acquired resistance. A patient with some acquired immunity, even if this by itself is insufficient to suppress totally the parasite, will require less supportive anti-malarial therapy. In general the greater the number of erythrocytic parasites a patient is exposed to before cure the more effective is the level of acquired immunity subsequently induced. Thus a large rapidly effective dose of an anti-malarial may in the long term be less beneficial than one or more smaller doses which prevents clinical malaria but allows a longer exposure to the parasite.

Anti-malarials are divided into four categories according to the stage in the life cycle they attack. Sporozoites are not killed by any anti-malarials. The causal prophylactics appear to kill early but not late liver stages and prevent erythrocytic infections. They are usually taken on a regular basis so that within the body there is always a minimal effective level of the anti-malarial present. Drugs which destroy all exo-erythrocytic forms are referred to as tissues schizontocides. Blood schizontocides act on the asexual erythrocytic parasites. Some anti-malarials affect the gametocytes, particularly the immature gametocytes and they are called gametocytocidal drugs. Finally some anti-malarials when taken up in a blood meal by the mosquito, will inhibit the development of the oocyst and thereby prevent the production of sporozoites: this anti-malarial activity is termed sporontocidal.

The commonly used anti-malarials are described briefly below:

Quinine is an alkaloid originally extracted from the bark of the Cinchona tree. Its history was described in Chapter 1. For nearly 300 years after its introduction to Europe quinine was the only available anti-malarial. It is now only used for the emergency treatment of falciparum malaria which fails to respond to chloroquine. Quinine is a bitter tasting blood schizonticide, and in the case of *P. vivax* and *P. malariae* also acts as a gametocytocide. The synthetic anti-malarials described below replaced quinine in the 1930s because they were more effective, less toxic and, in the case of *P. falciparum*, less frequently associated with blackwater fever.

Mepacrine, a 9-aminoacridine, was introduced in 1935 but is now considered obsolete. It is an effective blood schizonticide but among its disadvantages is the fact that it is laid down in the skin and the recipient turns a bright yellow!

Chloroquine and its very close relative *amodiaquine* are 4-aminoquinolines. Chloroquine was introduced in 1945 and is an excellent blood schizontocide and to *P. vivax*, *P. ovale* and *P. malariae* a gametocytocide. For the rapid control of acute malaria chloroquine is usually the drug of choice. It is rapidly absorbed but slowly excreted giving long term protection and is used for prophylactic and curative purposes. Since its activity is confined to the blood stages it will not destroy the persistent tissue forms of *P. vivax* and an individual infected with this parasite may suffer clinical attacks if he stops taking chloroquine.

Primaquine, first used in 1951, replaced the related pamaquine which was one of the first (1926) synthetic anti-malarials. Both are 8-aminoquinolines, destroy pre-erythrocytic stages and act as sporontocides. Both are toxic to the host, primaquine less so than pamaquine. The important role for primaquine is in the treatment of *P. vivax* infections where there may be persistent liver stages. The drug may induce haemolysis in G-6-PD deficient individuals (see Chapter 7).

Proguanil (introduced in 1948) a biguanide, and *pyrimethamine* (introduced 1952), a diaminopyrimidine, have similar activities. They destroy the early tissue stages, especially of *P. falciparum*, and hence are used as causal prophylactics. They also act as blood schizonticides, working more slowly than chloroquine, and as sporontocides. Both are relatively free of unpleasant side effects. Because of their mode of action these compounds are known as anti-folic drugs.

Sulphones such as dapsone (an anti-leprosy agent) and sulphonamides (e.g. sulphadiazine), both of which have pronounced anti-bacterial activity, have anti-malarial activity as blood schizonticides and are usually used in conjunction with other blood schizonticides, usually pyrimethamine.

9.2   Drug resistance

The menace of drug resistance to the attempts to rid areas of malaria and to ınaintain once malarious areas free of disease is referred to in Chapter 10. Drug resistance in the case of malaria has been defined by WHO as the ability of a strain of a malaria parasite to multiply or to survive in the presence of normal or above normal (i.e. up to maximum tolerated dose) concentrations of an anti-malarial. Drug resistance reported in the field is usually in relation to the asexual erythrocytic stage of *P. falciparum*. The sensitivity of a strain of *P. falciparum* to chloroquine and other anti-malarials was previously based on the course of the blood parasitaemia in patients given a standard form of the drug, e.g. 25 mg^{-1} kg of chloroquine. In the 1960s the finding that human malaria parasites would infect owl monkeys (*Aotus* sp.) allowed examination of the drug sensitivity of these parasites in these animals. More recently the drug sensitivity of *P. falciparum* has been assessed by observing the effect of the drug on the growth and multiplication of the parasite in *in vitro* cultures.

Resistance to the so-called anti-folate drugs, such as pyrimethamine and proguanil, has been recorded in all four species of human malarias, most frequently in South-East Asia and Africa, being first reported 25 years ago. Resistance to these causal prophylactics was not of major importance because they were not usually used for treating acute malaria. In contrast, resistance to the drug of choice for acute malaria, chloroquine, has only been described for *P. falciparum*. Such resistance was first observed in Columbia in 1961, not long after in Brazil, and subsequently in many parts of South-East Asia. Currently there are strong indications that chloroquine resistant strains of *P. falciparum* are present in the eastern half of Africa. Chloroquine resistance was itself alarming, but more serious was the finding that these chloroquine resistant strains were frequently also resistant to amodiaquine and mepacrine and worse still some were also less sensitive to quinine, which could usually be used to treat resistant *P. falciparum*. If this multiple resistance was to become widespread, particularly in India and Africa, the situation would arise in which the disease would be fought with an almost completely depleted armoury. Treatment of chloroquine resistant *P. falciparum* is attempted with a combination of quinine, a sulphonamide such as sulphadiazine, and pyrimethamine.

Drug-resistant strains presumably arise as a result of mutation and are selected for under widespread and frequent use of the drug in question. Genetic recombination between strains will lead to the dissemination of resistance. In the laboratory using rodent and avian malarias it has been very easy to develop strains resistant to the slow acting schizonticides such as pyrimethamine and proguanil but only with difficulty to the fast acting 4-aminoquinolines and quinine. How the drug resistant strains exert their resistance is not clear. The parasite could possibly be inactivating the drug – there is no evidence of this being the case. Secondly, a smaller amount of the drug may pass into the red cell and bind to the parasite; this has been demonstrated in chloroquine-resistant *P. falciparum* where it is thought that the parasite loses a high affinity chloroquine-binding site (see p. 50). A third possibility is that some metabolic pathway in the parasite is changed so that the effect of the drug is much reduced; this is thought to have happened in strains of parasites resistant to pyrimethamine, where a significant amount of the normally drug-sensitive enzyme dihydrofolate reductase appears in a changed form which does not bind the drug as well as the normal form of the enzyme.

9.3 Anti-malarial drug research

In the past the search for new anti-malarial drugs has gone in fits and starts, not least because the affluent countries with the resources for chemotherapeutic research no longer found malaria to be a serious indigenous health problem.

It is regrettable that the stimulus for determined efforts towards the development of new anti-malarials has been war. In World War I the German forces could no longer rely on their supply of quinine from the Far East and a consequence of this was the eventual development of pamaquine, mepacrine and later chloroquine. Similarly a shortage of quinine in World War II to the Allied Forces, stimulated research in the U.K. and the U.S.A. which produced primaquine, proguanil and pyrimethamine. More recently in the 1960s the U.S. involvement in South-East Asia, where chloroquine resistance became a major problem, led to the U.S. Defence Department sponsoring a major programme of research for new anti-malarials. Over 250 000 compounds were screened, out of which about half-a-dozen looked promising but to date only one compound, mefloquinine, is likely to become a commercially-available anti-malarial.

The development of a new anti-malarial is a long process. New compounds are synthesized. Some are related to existing drugs or to compounds which earlier screening studies had indicated might be promising. A few compounds are prepared on the basis of information available to the researcher about the biochemistry and physiology of the parasite: the so-called rational approach chemotherapy. The new compounds are screened for anti-malarial activity initially in mice against rodent malarias such as *P. berghei*, then against *P. falciparum* in owl monkeys and in *in vitro* culture. There are strains of *P. berghei* and *P. falciparum* available which are resistant to existing anti-malarials and hence it is possible to assess the potential value of new compounds for treating drug-resistant strains. Drug resistance, of course, is the main reason for searching for new anti-malarials. There are, however, dangers in using animal malarias or *in vitro* systems for screening compounds. It would be possible to miss compounds which have activity against human malarias but not against the animal malarias and to miss compounds which are active *in vivo* but not *in vitro*. Possibly in the latter case because the compounds have to be altered in the host to an active derivative. Proguanil, a powerful blood schizonticide in man, is poorly effective against *P. berghei* and would probably have been missed in a *P. berghei*/mouse-screening system. It is a long way from the discovery that a new compound has anti-malarial activity against drug-resistant strains in the primary screening systems to its commercial production. The new drug, particularly in the U.S.A. has to come through extremely stringent tests on its immediate and long term side effects on man (i.e. on children of all ages and adults, including pregnant women). Some of our older and still useful anti-malarials do have side effects and it is said that if they were introduced into the U.S.A. today their use would be prohibited. In addition, the new drug must be easily administered so that it can be used in mass chemotherapy campaigns. Finally it is worth stating the obvious. Drug companies have to be commercially viable. The people who need (new) anti-malarials, during peace time at least, invariably are those least able to buy them, and hence the development of new anti-malarials will almost certainly require support from public or private funds of which WHO is the most likely source.

9.4 How anti-malarials work

If we have a detailed understanding of the metabolic processes of a parasite protozoan it may be possible, by a systematic search, to identify which of these processes are disrupted by a drug which has activity against this protozoan. Unfortunately for many parasitic protozoa, including the malaria parasites, too little of the basic biochemistry of the parasite is known for this kind of study. Anti-malarials are known to affect energy metabolism, cofactor synthesis and nucleic-acid synthesis.

Starting with energy metabolism, it is thought that in the mammal the 8-aminoquinolines, e.g. primaquine, are broken down to a 5,6-quinoline diquinone, and analogue of ubiquinone which is found in the respiratory chain and hence may disrupt the respiratory chain of the malaria parasite. Under the electron microscope parasites treated with primaquine are seen to have swollen mitochondria.

Anti-malarials acting on membrane functions are not known. The antibacterial activity of the sulphonamides and sulphones is due to them, or compounds derived from them *in vivo*, acting as analogues of the growth factor *p*-amino benzoic acid (PABA). PABA is utilized in bacteria in the synthesis of dihydrofolate which is converted by the enzyme dihydrofolate reductase to tetrahydrofolate. Tetrahydrofolate is an important cofactor in a number of reactions including the interconversion of certain amino acids and the 'de novo' synthesis of some nucleotides. In bacteria the sulphonamides act by blocking the synthesis of dihydrofolate by inhibiting the enzyme dihydropteroate synthetase and it would appear that they have the same action on the malarial parasites which also need PABA as an essential growth factor in their diet (see Chapter 5). The reason why sulphonamides and sulphones act on the malaria parasite but not the host is that the parasite has to make its own dihydrofolate from PABA and guanosine triphosphate. The vertebrate host is able to utilize folates in the diet which are converted to dihydrofolate, and hence the host does not need the enzyme dihydropteroate synthetase. The anti-malarial 2,4-diaminopyrimidines such as pyrimethamine have already been referred to as 'anti-folates'. This is because their site of action is dihydrofolate reductase which catalyses the conversion of dihydrofolate to tetrahydrofolate. In this case the host has a similar enzyme but the enzyme in the parasite is very much more sensitive to the action of this drug than the vertebrate enzyme.

Quinine and chloroquine are thought to inhibit DNA and RNA synthesis, possibly because the drugs intercalate with DNA. Both these drugs, however, bind to DNA from any source. The reason why they selectively inhibit malaria parasite nucleic acid synthesis rather than that of the host is because the drug is concentrated in the parasitized red cells. Malaria parasites seem to have three binding sites for chloroquine and the drug can reach concentrations in the parasite 100–1000 times that in the surroundings medium.

In summary the need for new anti-malarials is pressing and if chloroquine resistance spreads further in the world, this need will become extremely urgent. There is much to learn about the biochemistry of a malaria parasite and the mode of action of anti-malarials and if more is known in these areas the development of new anti-malarials may be placed on a more rational basis and correspondingly proceed more rapidly.

10 Epidemiology and Eradication of Human Malaria

In order to unravel the complex epidemiological relationship found in malarious areas, and to understand the rationale behind the control measures that may be applied, we need a basic knowledge of the natural history of the *Anopheles* mosquito. The female *Anopheles* acts both as vector and as one of the hosts of the malaria parasite and in order for transmission to take place she must bite man at least twice and must live long enough (8–25 days depending on the species of malaria), at a suitable temperature, and relative humidity for the malaria parasite to complete its cycle of development within her.

10.1 Natural history of *Anopheles*

Anopheline mosquitoes are insects, Order Diptera, Sub-order Nematocera, and Genus *Anopheles* . There are approximately 400 species of *Anopheles* described but of these only about 60 species are major vectors of malaria. *Anopheles* mosquitoes, although mainly tropical and subtropical insects, are also found in the temperate areas and even the Arctic.

The male *Anopheles* feeds on nectar and fruit juices whereas the female takes both these plant products and blood. Her mouthparts are adapted to pierce the skin and are long and slender enough to imbibe blood directly from skin capillaries. A mosquito, if undisturbed, will be replete with blood within a few minutes during which she may have taken up 5.0 μl of blood.

The life cycle of the mosquito consists of four phases: egg, larva, pupa and adult. The emerging adult mosquitoes copulate within a day or so, usually in flight and after one or two blood meals the first batch of several hundred eggs are laid, singly, at the breeding site. The female may lay several batches of eggs during her life, each batch being preceded by a blood meal and with an interval between each oviposition (egg-laying) of 2–3 days. The interval between each oviposition is known as the gonotrophic cycle. The eggs, about 500 μm long and equipped with floats, hatch within 2–3 days, releasing the larvae into the water. The larvae feed at, and usually lie parallel to, the surface. After 3 moults over a few days, the larvae transform into the non-feeding pupae. Within the pupae, over a period of 2–4 days, metamorphosis takes place, culminating in the emergence of the adults. Males usually emerge before the females. The period required for the newly laid egg to become an adult mosquito depends on the species and the conditions, particularly temperature. *A. gambiae* may complete the cycle in about 7 days at 30°C but at 20°C may take 3 times as long. A transient puddle may therefore last long enough for a batch of eggs to complete development. Of crucial importance to the parasite is how long its dipterous vector survives: the average life span of the females of some species may be almost a month.

Control of malaria revolves around attacks on the vector and the parasite. The attacks on the vector are aimed at the larva and the adult. In order to reduce the number of larvae several measures can be employed, all of which to some degree depend on a knowledge of the kind of breeding sites the mosquitoes frequent. It is preferable to remove the breeding sites altogether but if this is not possible they are made inhospitable to the female mosquito and the larvae. The factors which influence the choice of breeding site include salinity, temperature, amount of light and shade, and the amount of organic materials in the water. Apart from large expanses of open water and clean edged tanks and reservoirs, mosquitoes will breed in anything containing water. Larval habitats, temporary and permanent, are grouped under broad headings.

(*i*)   Standing fresh water – swamps, paddy fields, wells.

(*ii*) Temporary fresh water – rain water pools in footprints, cart-tracks and similar depressions.

(*iii*) Slowly running water – edges of streams, irrigation channels, canals, rivers, ditches.

(*iv*) Container habitats – leaf axils, tins, tyres, cisterns.

(*v*)   Brackish water – tidal swamps, marshes.

The behaviour of the adult female *Anopheles* is related to whether it has a role as a vector of malaria or not: as a vector it has to take at least two blood meals from man, the first from a person carrying the parasite. Feeding takes place between dusk and dawn, each species having a preferred biting period. (During the day some species may feed in dark gloomy situations.) Given a choice, each species takes blood from a limited range of host species, some preferring animals (zoophilic) and others man (anthrophilic). How the insect locates its prey is not fully understood but involves a combination of stimuli such as sight and smell and an ability to move up carbon dioxide gradients. The chemical stimuli emanating from the host are collectively known as the attractant plume. The mosquito's search flight brings it into contact with this. The final approach is upwind.

A replete mosquito needs to rest so that the volume of the blood meal can be reduced and digestion commence. Some rest on the walls and ceilings of the house in which they fed, while others prefer to rest outside human habitation. Mosquitoes have been classfied according to their resting habits into *endophilic*, mosquitoes which remain in human habitation for a good proportion of their lifetime, and *exophilic*, those largely found outside human habitation although they may feed on man within his dwellings.

10.2   Epidemiology of malaria

First we will list some of the conditions which have to be met for transmission to occur within a community. The malaria parasite is probably already within the community but occasionally it may be introduced from outside in the vertebrate or insect host. There must be a proportion of the population which is susceptible to infection and in whom gametocytes can develop. There must be sufficient numbers of vector(s) which have a preference for human blood or are in a situation where their preferred host is absent, and there is little alternative but to feed on man. The vectors must feed on man with the requisite frequency. A large enough proportion of the vectors must survive long enough for the parasite to complete its sporogonic cycle and the environmental temperature and relative humidity must suit both mosquito and *Plasmodium*. Having set out these basic requirements for transmission it has to be said that the precise demands of the different species of *Plasmodium* in man are not the same. For example, the longevity of *P. malariae* infections and the relapse nature of some *P. vivax* infections may mean that there can be considerable periods when vector and parasite do not make contact but transmission over a long period can be maintained.

The environmental conditions affect both vector and parasite. Temperature should be between 18 and 30°C and relative humidity 60–70% or above. Malaria is dependent on rainfall, partly by providing breeding habitats and also by maintaining relative humidity which increases the longevity of the mosquitoes. The rainy season in many tropical localities is associated with malaria, its onset being accompanied by a rapid rise in the numbers of mosquitoes and the relative humidity. Too much rain, however, can be bad for mosquitoes, slowly running streams becoming gushing torrents which flush out the larvae and pupae from their shelter along the banks. In contrast, and paradoxically, there have been occasions when drought precipitates favourable conditions for malaria. For example, in Sri Lanka in 1934 a failure of the monsoon led to the rivers drying up and shallow pools forming where once there was a steady flow of water. These pools presented ideal breeding sites for *A. culicifacies*, the main vector of malaria in Sri Lanka.

Although malaria is widespread in the world the degree to which each individual community is affected by malaria at any one time and in any one year may vary. The extent of malaria in a region is categorized by malariologists as endemic or epidemic.

In the *endemic* situation the incidence of malaria is fairly constant over a period of successive years. Endemic malaria is subdivided into hypo-endemic (little transmission, spleen rate (see later) in children 2–9 years less than 10%), meso-endemic (transmission rate variable, spleen rate in children 2–9 years 11–50%), hyper-endemic (intense but seasonal transmission, spleen rate in children 2–9 years greater than 50% and in adults greater than 25%), and holo-endemic (perennial extensive transmission, spleen rate in children 2–9 years greater than 75% and in adults low). Where malaria is hyper- or holo-endemic the situation is said to be stable, immunity because of frequent re-infection being high in all but the babies and children up to the age of 5 years. In the unstable situation, from year to year the amount of transmission varies and the immunity throughout the population, young and old. is low.

In the *epidemic* situation there is a slow and then rapid increase in the incidence of infection, which occurs sporadically. Epidemics occur when a population has low level of immunity, either the indigenous population or in some cases an immigrant population, a labour force or an army for example, and this vulnerable population is exposed to increased numbers of vectors carrying the malaria parasites. The increased exposure to infected mosquitoes may simply be the result of an increase in the mosquito population. Alternatively mosquito numbers may not change but an introduction of gametocyte carriers into the area from outside will lead to an increase in the number of infected mosquitoes.

A third possibility is that a zoophilic mosquito may become anthrophilic if suddenly deprived of its usual source of food. This happened in Italy just after the Second World War when there were few cattle and other livestock to feed on and the mosquitoes had to feed on man.

10.2   The epidemiology of malaria

The epidemiology of malaria has been put onto a quantitative basis, the major efforts in this direction being by the late Professor G. MacDonald in his book *The Epidemiology and Control of Malaria*. The numerous factors which determine the rate of transmission and the incidence of malaria were measured and their relationships expressed mathematically. It is beyond the scope of this book to do other than indicate the kind of measurements and how they were made. The incidence of malaria in a population is assessed by examination of stained blood smears, by determining the spleen rate and by serological tests which indicate the incidence and level of anti-malarial antibodies. The spleen enlarges during malaria and this enlargement can be detected and semiquantified by palpation. The spleen rate simply means the proportion of the population with an enlarged spleen. For the vector it is possible to determine (*i*) their density in relation to man (by, for example, using traps, live bait, or spraying and collecting the dead mosquitoes), (*ii*) the life expectancy or daily survival rate (examination of the ovaries of mosquitoes can give a reasonable estimate of the mosquito's age providing the length of the gonotrophic cycle is known), (*iii*) the source of the blood meal (using the serological precipitin test) and the frequency of bites on man, (*iv*) the length of the sporogonic cycle in the vector at the prevailing temperature and (*v*) the proportion of mosquitoes carrying malaria parasites as infective sporozoites (by examining the mosquito's salivary glands and mid-gut under the microscope). Using data of this kind it is possible to express mathematically the so-called vectorial capacity of the vector population, i.e. the predicted infective bites of man per case of malaria each day, and the basic reproduction rate of the parasite, i.e. the predicted new cases of malaria derived from a single infected person.

10.3   Control of malaria

The methods used for reducing the incidence of malaria are designed to interrupt the cycle of the parasite between its two hosts and to reduce the number of mosquitoes. In the early part of this century it was soon realised that every malarious area needs individual attention in order to identify which mosquitoes are vectors, and their breeding and biting habits and then to tailor a programme of control accordingly.

If the infected mosquito is prevented from feeding on man infection cannot take place. Measures to bring this about include bed-nets, mosquito screens, protective clothing and the application of insect repellants to the exposed skin. Houses should be situated away from sites frequented by mosquitoes. Should infected mosquitoes bite man the administration of anti-malarial compounds (see Chapter 9) can either prevent infection occuring or be used to eliminate an established infection and reduce the infectivity of gametocytes to other vectors.

The attack on the mosquito itself can be on a number of fronts. First the number of breeding sites can be reduced by filling in or emptying water-holding depressions and containers. This was one of the earliest control methods advocated by Ross amongst others. However, construction of irrigation canals, the extension of rice paddies and the clearing of jungle to allow in sunlight are all examples of developments to promote human well-being which incidentally increase the available breeding sites to particular species of vectors with a consequent increase in malaria. Anti-larval methods include the spraying of oil or Paris green onto the water surface in the breeding sites. The film of oil asphyxiates and poisons the larvae, and the Paris green (copper acetic arsensite), which is a fine green powder, is ingested and poisons them. The intermittent drying out or flushing of water courses in which the flow can be managed, such as irrigation channels, can reduce the numbers of larvae. Larvivorous fish, such as the guppy and minnows, have also been successfully used to reduce larval numbers.

Since 1945, with the advent of the insecticide DDT (dichloro diphenyl trichloroethane), the main focus of attack has been on the adult mosquito by house-spraying. The rationale is simple. The engorged endophilic mosquito rests in some dark position in the house and if that position has previously been sprayed with a residual insecticide the vector is killed before she can transmit the parasite. During the course of a fortnight a female mosquito may feed half a dozen times and in seeking a resting place on each occasion the chances are high of her coming into contact with the insecticide. Spraying usually does not eliminate the vector but by claiming a daily mortality of up to 50% it does reduce the life expectancy within the population to a level when transmission could not take place. Spraying of houses is easier to organize, easier to train personnel to carry out, and more easily effected on a countrywide basis than anti-larval measures. House spraying with DDT was hugely successful. *A. funestus*, for example, disappeared from Mauritius almost immediately. DDT is very persistent, two sprayings each year being sufficient, it is cheap and when first introduced it was thought to be non-toxic to higher animals. Other organochlorines such as HCH (hexachlorocyclohexane) and dieldrin, introduced around the same time as DDT, were effective but had to be applied more frequently. Pyrethrum, a natural insecticide extracted from the dried flowers of *Chrysanthemum cinerariaefolium*, is effective but is rapidly inactivated by sunlight, and hence it is not persistent and requires repeated applications

The early success with DDT and the other organochlorines created such optimism that in 1957 WHO thought malaria eradication from the world possible. In the last decade, however, these particular insecticides have fallen out of favour to some degree. First their persistence, which makes them such effective insecticides, has brought them into trouble as environmental pollutants, progressively concentrating in animals up the food chains and in so doing, proving harmful to wild life. Secondly, resistance to them by the mosquito has become more widespread. In 1946 two species of *Anopheles* were resistant to DDT. Contrast this with the situation in 1976 when 3 species were resistant to DDT only, 21 species to DDT and dieldrin and 42 species to dieldrin. In one part of the world the same species of *Anopheles* may have members resistant to DDT but in another part sensitive forms only. Resistance to dieldrin developed more rapidly than DDT. The rate at which resistant populations of mosquitoes emerged was speeded up by the widespread use of these insecticides in agriculture to control pests on crops such as cotton. DDT ran off from agricultural land into the mosquitoes' breeding areas.

For spraying there are alternative insecticides to the organochlorines such as the organophosphorous compounds (e.g. malathion), carbonates (e.g. propoxur), and the synthetic pyrethrum-like compounds, the pyrethroids, which do have residual activity. All these, however, also suffer from the problem of the vector developing resistance to them. In 1976 the majority of vectors for malaria were known to be resistant to at least one insecticide. DDT is much cheaper than the alternatives. For example in 1977 1 t of DDT cost approximately \$950 whereas 1 t of malathion was \$1350. Moreover, because malathion had to be sprayed more frequently it was estimated that in 1977 the cost of DDT to protect 1 million people was \$279 000 and of malathion \$1 188 000.

Possible new approaches to mosquito control are only at the developmental stage. These include genetic control, e.g. using the sterile male technique in which the fecundity of the population is reduced by releasing sterile males into it, and the introduction of pathogens harmful to mosquitoes such as bacteria (*Bacillus sphaericus*), protozoa (*Nosema*), fungi (*Coelomyces*) and nematodes.

10.4   Eradication

In 1955 the Eighth World Assembly adopted a global eradication programme. Two years later WHO took over the task of coordinating the efforts towards the goal of eradication. Within malarious areas malaria eradication programmes consist of four phases, lasting 8 or more years in total. During the one or two years of the first or preparatory phase the ground work is done. The area is surveyed, the staff trained and the size of problem identified. In the second or attack phase the mosquito vectors are attacked by house-spraying and other measures. The aim is to provide a complete attack on the vector. At the same time anti-malarial drugs may be distributed when necessary. The attack phase may last four years or more, during which time the degree of transmission and the number of people infected with malaria should decline. When less than 1 in 10 000 is positive for parasites the programme moves into the third or consolidation phase, a period of surveillance and action if any cases are detected. The final phase, the maintenance phase, comes into operation if during the three preceding years there were no indigenous cases of malaria. The maintenance phase is one of continual vigilance.

What has been achieved by these coordinated programmes to alleviate the considerable burden levied by malaria? By the end of 1976 (WHO figures), of the estimated 2048 million people living in the originally malarious areas of the world, 436 million were residing in parts of the world which were them thought to be malaria free, 1250 million in areas where control and eradication measures were underway, but 352 million were still in areas where no specific anti-malarial measures were operative. Over the past 20 years or so, the global anti-malaria programme has provided protection for an increasing number of people. In 1960 it was estimated that 2.5 million people died from malaria each year. The present figure is thought to be about half this. In India in 1950 three quarters of a million people died from malaria. In 1965 this figure was reduced to 1500 deaths, a considerable achievement. Malaria has been eliminated from the whole of Europe, parts of the Middle East, most of North America, most of the Caribbean, parts of South America, much of the Far East and Australia. These achievements, however, are tempered by the fact that malaria is still endemic over much of the tropics. Tropical Africa for example is almost as malarious to the indigenous population as it ever was with the exception of some of the larger towns which enjoy some limited mosquito control measures. Worse still is that some of the early gains have been, or are being, lost. In India, which was the subject of the biggest single eradication programme in a developing country, the number of cases in the 1960s was reduced to a few 10 000s: in 1976 it was estimated that there were 10 million. Resurgences have also occurred in other parts of Asia, in Central and South America and Turkey.

There are many reasons why malaria remains such a major threat to the health and the socio-economic development of many developing countries (one writer has suggested that malaria now poses a threat on the same scale as it did in the 1950s). The existing anti-malarial measures may be inadequate – the result of mosquitoes being resistant to insecticides, parasites resistant to anti-malarials (particularly *P. falciparum* resistence to chloroquine), anti-mosquito measures being poorly applied, or simply that the present methods, which have been effective in one area, are unsuitable for the particular local conditions of another area. For example, if the vectors in one rural area are exophilic, reducing the effectiveness of house-spraying and at the same time anti-larval measures are difficult to implement. The disruptive effects of political unrest, civil war, invasion and declining economies are self-evident and that such conditions prevail in many parts of the world are well known.

The situation therefore is not good. Indeed it has been said that if chloroquine resistant *P. falciparum* spreads into India, and from Kenya and Ethiopia into other parts of Africa a major health catastrophe could occur. To quote M. Farid 'The malaria dragon is now with us, and will teach us still many lessons and inflict catastrophes; but we can avoid these catastrophes if we have the foresight, the knowledge of the magnitude of its striking power, and the determination to stand strong and united against it'.

Further Reading

BRUCE-CHWATT, L. J. (1980). *Essential Malariology*. Heinemann, London.

COHEN, S. and WARREN, K.S. (eds) (1982). *Immunology of Parasitic Infections*. Blackwell, Oxford.

COHEN, S. (ed.) (1982). Malaria. *British Medical Bulletin*, Churchill Livingstone, Edinburgh, **38**, 115–218.

GARNHAM, P. C. C. (1966). *Malaria Parasites and Other Haemosporidia*. Blackwell, Oxford.

GUTTERIDGE, W. E. and COOMBS, G. H. (1977). *Biochemistry of Parasitic Protozoa*. MacMillian, London.

HARRISON, G. (1978). *Mosquitoes, Malaria and Men: A History of the Hostilities Since 1880*. John Murray, London.

KILLICK-KENDRICK, R. and PETERS, W. (eds) (1978). *Rodent Malaria*. Academic Press, New York and London.

KREIER, J. P. (ed.) (1977). *Parasitic Protozoa*. 4 volumes. Academic Press, New York and London.

Index